NO GALLBLADDER DIET COOKBOOK

Guide to Transform Your Metabolism Including Nutritional Recipes for Optimal Well-being

TABLE OF CONTENTS

CHAPTER 1: INTRODUCTION

A place where flavors dance and gastronomic delights develop sits at the core of culinary inquiry. Welcome to the "NO Gallbladder Diet Cookbook" a culinary guide for people who are navigating the unique journey of life without a gallbladder. Set out on a scrumptious journey where each recipe is a symphony of taste and health designed to embrace the intricacies of a gallbladder-friendly lifestyle. Join us as we reimagine the art of cooking without compromise, demonstrating that bright, tasty meals can coexist with your health. This cookbook is more than just a compilation of recipes; it is a celebration of the delightful union of flavor and mindful eating. Prepare to savor each page as we welcome you to a world where gastronomic delight meets the wisdom of a NO gallbladder diet.

UNDERSTANDING THE NO GALLBLADDER DIET

1. Fat Management: Without the gallbladder to store bile, controlling fat intake is critical for avoiding digestive problems. It is beneficial to use lean sources and fewer quantities.
2. Bile Release: After gallbladder removal bile which is necessary for fat breakdown, is secreted more steadily. Eating smaller, more evenly distributed meals helps to facilitate this altered bile flow.
3. Low-Fat Foods: Prioritizing low-fat foods, such as lean proteins, fruits and vegetables reduces digestive stress.
4. Nutritional Balance: Eating a well-balanced diet promotes optimal nutrient uptake. The combination of proteins, carbs and good fats promotes general health.
5. Fiber for Digestive Health: Consuming fiber-rich foods aids digestion and prevents constipation which is a typical post-surgery problem.
6. Importance of Hydration: Staying hydrated is critical for digestion and general health. It also aids in the prevention of problems such as gallstone formation.

7. Individualized Approach: Following gallbladder ectomy, each person may react differently to various meals. It is critical to monitor and adjust the diet based on individual responses.

8. Food Gradual Inclusion: Introducing new meals gradually allows the body to adjust and aids in the identification of any specific triggers or intolerances.

IMPORTANCE OF DIETARY ADJUSTMENTS

1. Fat Digestion: Because the gallbladder holds bile, removing it can impair fat digestion. Choosing low-fat foods helps to minimize discomfort and improves digestion.

2. Smaller More Frequent Meals: Eating smaller more frequent meals can help with digestion because the body copes better with less bile availability.

3. Fiber consumption supports regular bowel movements, preventing constipation which is a typical problem following gallbladder removal.

4. Hydration: Staying hydrated aids digestion and helps to prevent issues such as gallstones.

5. Balanced Nutrition: Including lean proteins, entire grains and plenty of fruits and vegetables in a balanced diet ensures that total nutritional demands are met.

6. Identifying and avoiding foods that may cause digestive discomfort such as fried or fatty foods might improve post-surgery well-being.

7. Gradual introductions of new meals allow the body to adjust and aid in the identification of specific triggers or intolerances.

8. Monitoring Symptoms: Paying attention to digestive symptoms and changing the diet as needed guarantees personalized and successful post-gallbladder removal care.

CHAPTER 2: OVERVIEW OF THE DIGESTIVE PROCESS

1. The process starts with the intake of food through the mouth.
2. Mastication (chewing): Teeth break down food into smaller bits, increasing the surface area for enzymes to work on.
3. Salivary Enzymes: Saliva which contains enzymes such as amylase, begins to break down carbs into simpler sugars.
4. Swallowing: The chewed food is swallowed and goes down the esophagus to the stomach via peristalsis.
5. Stomach: Gastric juices, such as hydrochloric acid and enzymes further break down the meal into chyme, a semi-liquid material.
6. Small Intestine: The small intestine is responsible for the majority of digestion and nutrition absorption. Fats, proteins and carbohydrates are broken down by pancreatic enzymes bile from the liver, and intestinal enzymes.
7. Nutrient absorption occurs when nutrients pass past the small intestine's walls into the bloodstream and are delivered to cells throughout the body.
8. Water and electrolytes are absorbed from the remaining indigestible material resulting in feces.
9. Feces pass into the colon where microorganisms aid in fermentation creating various vitamins and gases.
10. Rectum and Anus: Feces are retained in the rectum until they are eliminated via the anus.

FOODS TO AVOID AND INCLUDE

Foods to Avoid on a Gallbladder-Free Diet:

1. High-Fat Foods: Without the gallbladder, fried foods, fatty cuts of meat and rich sauces might be difficult to digest.
2. Spices: Spices can cause intestinal pain and should be limited or avoided.

3. Full-fat dairy products may be more difficult to digest. Choose low-fat or lactose-free options.
4. Highly processed and oily foods can contribute to digestive problems.
5. Foods that produce gas: Some people may need to reduce gas-producing foods such as beans, cabbage and carbonated beverages.
6. Certain veggies: Cruciferous veggies (such as broccoli and cauliflower) might be difficult for certain people to digest; consider boiling them to make them more digestible.

Foods to Eat If You Don't Have a Gallbladder:

1. Skinless poultry, fish, lean cuts of meat and plant-based protein sources like tofu are also good options.
2. Low-Fat Dairy: To aid digestion, choose low-fat or fat-free dairy products.
3. Fruits and Vegetables: For critical vitamins and minerals, eat a range of colorful fruits and vegetables.
4. Whole Grains: Include whole grains like brown rice, quinoa and oats in your diet for fiber and long-lasting energy.
5. Healthy Fats: Consume healthy fats in moderation such as avocados, olive oil and almonds.
6. Drink plenty of water to aid digestion and prevent dehydration.
7. Smaller, More Frequent Meals: Eating smaller, more frequent meals can aid digestion.

STAYING ACTIVE AND MAINTAINING A HEALTHY WEIGHT

1. Regular Exercise: For cardiovascular health and muscle strength incorporate a combination of aerobic workouts (such as walking, running or cycling) and strength training into your programme.
2. Consistency is essential: Aim for at least 150 minutes of moderate-intensity activity per week or 75 minutes of vigorous-intensity exercise per week as well as muscle-strengthening exercises on two or more days each week.

3. Find Enjoyable Activities: Choose physical activities that you enjoy in order to make fitness a habit.

4. Focus on a well-balanced diet that includes a variety of nutrients. Fruits, vegetables, whole grains, lean meats and healthy fats should all be included.

5. Control your portion amounts to avoid overeating and maintain a healthy weight.

6. Hydration: Drink enough water every day to improve your general health and digestion.

7. Adequate Sleep: Get enough quality sleep because a lack of sleep can affect your weight and overall well-being.

8. Set Realistic Goals: To stay motivated and measure your progress, set realistic and achievable fitness and weight goals.

9. Small modifications to your everyday routine such as taking the stairs, walking more or standing instead of sitting can make a big difference.

10. Regular Health Examinations: Schedule regular health checks to monitor your weight, examine your exercise levels and treat any new health concerns.

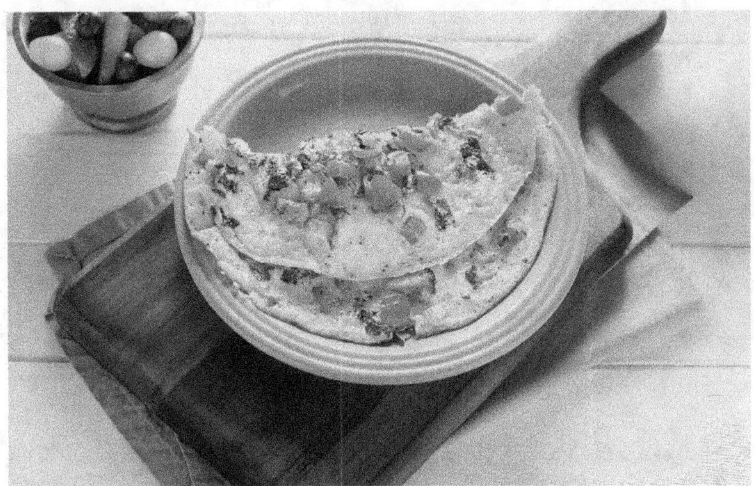

Vegetable Omelet:

Ingredients:

- 3 large eggs
- 1/4 cup milk
- Salt and pepper to taste
- 1 tablespoon olive oil
- 1/4 cup diced bell peppers (any color)
- 1/4 cup diced onions
- 1/4 cup diced tomatoes
- 1/4 cup chopped spinach
- 1/4 cup grated cheese (optional)

Instructions:

1. Crack the eggs into a bowl, add milk, salt and pepper. Whisk until well combined.

2. Heat olive oil in a non-stick skillet over medium heat.

3. Add diced bell peppers and onions to the skillet. Sauté until they soften.

4. Add tomatoes and chopped spinach. Cook until the spinach wilts and the tomatoes soften.

5. Pour the whisked eggs over the vegetables in the skillet.

6. Allow the eggs to set around the edges, then gently lift them with a spatula to let the uncooked eggs flow underneath.

7. Once the omelet is mostly set but still slightly runny on top, sprinkle grated cheese if using.

8. Carefully fold the omelet in half using the spatula.

9. Cook for an additional 1-2 minutes until the cheese melts and the omelet is cooked through.

10. Slide the vegetable omelet onto a plate, cut in half if desired and serve hot.

Greek Yogurt Parfait:

Ingredients:

- 1 cup Greek yogurt
- 2 tablespoons honey or maple syrup
- 1/2 cup granola
- 1/2 cup mixed berries (strawberries, blueberries, raspberries)
- 1 tablespoon chopped nuts (almonds, walnuts or your preference)
- Fresh mint leaves for garnish (optional)

Instructions:

1. In a bowl, mix Greek yogurt with honey or maple syrup until well combined.

2. In serving glasses or bowls, start layering the parfait. Begin with a spoonful of the sweetened Greek yogurt.

3. Add a layer of granola on top of the yogurt.

4. Sprinkle a layer of mixed berries over the granola.

5. Repeat the layers until the glass or bowl is filled, ending with a final layer of berries on top.

6. Sprinkle chopped nuts over the berry layer for added crunch and flavor.

7. Optionally, garnish with fresh mint leaves for a burst of freshness.

8. Serve immediately and enjoy your delicious Greek Yogurt Parfait!

Oatmeal with Fruit:

Ingredients:

- 1/2 cup rolled oats
- 1 cup milk (dairy or plant-based)
- 1/2 cup water
- Pinch of salt
- 1/2 teaspoon vanilla extract
- 1 banana, sliced
- 1/2 cup berries (strawberries, blueberries or your choice)
- 1 tablespoon honey or maple syrup
- Optional toppings: chopped nuts, seeds or shredded coconut

Instructions:

1. In a saucepan, combine rolled oats, milk, water and a pinch of salt.

2. Bring the mixture to a gentle boil over medium heat, then reduce heat to low.

3. Simmer the oats, stirring occasionally, until they reach your desired consistency (usually 5-7 minutes).

4. Stir in vanilla extract for added flavor.

5. Once the oatmeal is cooked, transfer it to a bowl.

6. Top the oatmeal with sliced bananas, berries and any additional toppings you prefer.

7. Drizzle honey or maple syrup over the fruits for sweetness.

8. Give it a gentle stir to combine the flavors.

9. Serve warm and enjoy your nutritious oatmeal with a burst of fruity goodness.

Smoothie Bowl:

Ingredients:

- 1 frozen banana, sliced
- 1 cup frozen mixed berries (strawberries, blueberries, raspberries)
- 1/2 cup Greek yogurt
- 1/2 cup milk (dairy or plant-based)
- 1 tablespoon honey or maple syrup (optional for sweetness)
- Toppings: sliced fruits, granola, chia seeds, shredded coconut, nuts

Instructions:

1. In a blender, combine frozen banana slices, frozen berries, Greek yogurt and milk.
2. Blend until smooth and creamy. Add honey or maple syrup if extra sweetness is desired.
3. Pour the smoothie into a bowl.
4. Arrange your favorite toppings on the smoothie surface. Get creative with a variety of textures and flavors.
5. Enjoy your vibrant and nutritious smoothie bowl with a spoon!

Quinoa Breakfast Bowl:

Ingredients:

- 1/2 cup quinoa, rinsed
- 1 cup milk (dairy or plant-based)
- 1/2 teaspoon vanilla extract
- 1 tablespoon honey or maple syrup
- 1/2 cup sliced fresh fruits (bananas, berries or your choice)
- 1 tablespoon chopped nuts (almonds, walnuts or your preference)
- 1 tablespoon seeds (chia seeds, flaxseeds or pumpkin seeds)
- Optional: Greek yogurt for extra creaminess

Instructions:

1. Rinse quinoa under cold water.

2. In a saucepan, combine quinoa, milk and vanilla extract.

3. Bring the mixture to a boil, then reduce heat to low, cover, and simmer for about 15 minutes or until quinoa is cooked and liquid is absorbed.

4. Stir in honey or maple syrup for sweetness.

5. Once quinoa is cooked, transfer it to a bowl.

6. Top the quinoa with sliced fresh fruits, chopped nuts and seeds.

7. Optionally, add a dollop of Greek yogurt for creaminess.

8. Drizzle a bit more honey or maple syrup if desired.

9. Give it a gentle stir to combine the flavors.

10. Enjoy your nutritious and satisfying quinoa breakfast bowl!

Egg and Spinach Breakfast Wrap:

Ingredients:

- 1 large tortilla or wrap
- 2 large eggs
- 1 cup fresh spinach leaves, chopped
- 1/4 cup diced tomatoes
- 1/4 cup shredded cheese (cheddar, mozzarella, or your choice)
- Salt and pepper to taste
- 1 tablespoon olive oil or cooking spray
- Optional toppings: salsa, avocado slices, hot sauce

Instructions:

1. In a bowl, beat the eggs and season with salt and pepper.

2. Heat olive oil in a skillet over medium heat.

3. Add chopped spinach to the skillet and sauté until wilted.

4. Push the spinach to the side and pour the beaten eggs into the skillet.

5. Scramble the eggs, incorporating the spinach as they cook.

6. When the eggs are almost set, add diced tomatoes and shredded cheese. Mix until the cheese is melted and eggs are fully cooked.

7. Warm the tortilla in a separate pan or microwave.

8. Spoon the egg and spinach mixture onto the center of the tortilla.

9. Add optional toppings like salsa, avocado slices, or hot sauce.

10. Fold the sides of the tortilla over the filling, creating a wrap.

Chia Seed Pudding:

Ingredients:

- 1/4 cup chia seeds
- 1 cup milk (dairy or plant-based)
- 1 tablespoon honey or maple syrup
- 1/2 teaspoon vanilla extract
- Optional toppings: fresh berries, sliced fruits, nuts, shredded coconut

Instructions:

1. In a bowl, combine chia seeds, milk, honey or maple syrup, and vanilla extract.

2. Whisk the mixture thoroughly to ensure the chia seeds are well dispersed.

3. Let the mixture sit for about 5 minutes, then whisk again to prevent clumping.

4. Cover the bowl and refrigerate for at least 2 hours or overnight to allow the chia seeds to absorb the liquid and form a pudding-like consistency.

5. After refrigeration, give the chia pudding a good stir.

6. Spoon the chia seed pudding into serving glasses or bowls.

7. Top with your favorite toppings such as fresh berries, sliced fruits, nuts, or shredded coconut.

8. Drizzle a bit more honey or maple syrup if desired.

9. Enjoy your creamy and nutritious Chia Seed Pudding as a delightful breakfast or snack.

Cottage Cheese with Pineapple:

Ingredients:

- 1 cup cottage cheese

- 1 cup fresh pineapple chunks (or canned pineapple tidbits, drained)
- 1 tablespoon honey or maple syrup (optional, for added sweetness)
- 1/4 cup chopped mint leaves (optional, for garnish)

Instructions:

1. In a bowl, combine cottage cheese and fresh pineapple chunks.
2. If desired, drizzle honey or maple syrup over the mixture for added sweetness.
3. Gently toss the ingredients together until well combined.
4. Allow the flavors to meld for a few minutes.
5. Optionally, sprinkle chopped mint leaves over the top for a refreshing garnish.
6. Serve immediately and enjoy this simple and nutritious Cottage Cheese with Pineapple.

Sweet Potato Hash:

Ingredients:

- 2 medium-sized sweet potatoes, peeled and diced
- 1 bell pepper, diced
- 1 onion, diced
- 2 cloves garlic, minced
- 2 tablespoons olive oil
- 1 teaspoon smoked paprika
- 1/2 teaspoon cumin
- Salt and pepper to taste
- Fresh parsley or cilantro for garnish (optional)
- Eggs (optional, for serving on top)

Instructions:

1. Heat olive oil in a large skillet over medium heat.
2. Add diced sweet potatoes to the skillet and cook for about 5 minutes, stirring occasionally.

3. Add diced bell pepper and onion to the skillet. Continue cooking until the sweet potatoes are tender and the vegetables are slightly caramelized.
4. Stir in minced garlic, smoked paprika, cumin, salt, and pepper. Cook for an additional 2-3 minutes to allow the flavors to meld.
5. If desired, make wells in the hash with a spoon and crack eggs into the wells. Cover the skillet and cook until the eggs are cooked to your liking.
6. Garnish with fresh parsley or cilantro if desired.
7. Serve the Sweet Potato Hash on its own or with a side of eggs for a hearty and flavorful breakfast or brunch.

Whole Grain Toast with Avocado:

Ingredients:

- 2 slices of whole grain bread
- 1 ripe avocado
- Lemon juice (optional, to prevent avocado from browning)
- Salt and pepper to taste
- Red pepper flakes (optional, for added spice)
- Toasted sesame seeds or everything bagel seasoning (optional, for extra flavor)

Instructions:

1. Toast the whole grain bread slices to your desired level of crispiness.
2. While the bread is toasting, cut the avocado in half, remove the pit, and scoop the flesh into a bowl.
3. Mash the avocado with a fork until it reaches your preferred consistency.
4. If you like, add a squeeze of lemon juice to the mashed avocado to prevent browning. Mix well.
5. Season the mashed avocado with salt and pepper to taste. Add red pepper flakes for a touch of spice if desired.
6. Once the bread is toasted, spread the mashed avocado evenly over each slice.

7. Optionally, sprinkle toasted sesame seeds or everything bagel seasoning on top for extra flavor.

8. Serve immediately and savor the delicious and nutritious Whole Grain Toast with Avocado.

Buckwheat Pancakes:

Ingredients:

- 1 cup buckwheat flour
- 1 tablespoon sugar
- 1 teaspoon baking powder
- 1/2 teaspoon baking soda
- 1/4 teaspoon salt
- 1 cup buttermilk
- 1 large egg
- 2 tablespoons melted butter or oil
- Optional: 1/2 teaspoon vanilla extract
- Cooking spray or additional butter for greasing the pan

Instructions:

1. In a large bowl, whisk together buckwheat flour, sugar, baking powder, baking soda, and salt.

2. In a separate bowl, whisk together buttermilk, egg, melted butter or oil, and vanilla extract if using.

3. Pour the wet ingredients into the dry ingredients and stir until just combined. Be careful not to overmix; a few lumps are okay.

4. Let the batter rest for 10-15 minutes to allow the buckwheat flour to absorb the liquid.

5. Heat a griddle or non-stick skillet over medium heat. Lightly grease with cooking spray or butter.

6. Pour 1/4 cup portions of batter onto the hot griddle for each pancake.

7. Cook until bubbles form on the surface of the pancake, then flip and cook the other side until golden brown.

8. Repeat until all the batter is used, adjusting heat as needed.

9. Serve the buckwheat pancakes warm, topped with your favorite toppings like maple syrup, fresh berries, or a dollop of yogurt.

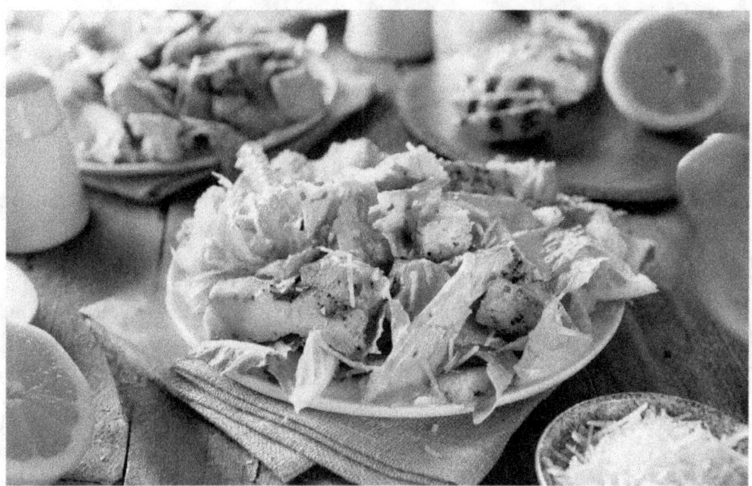

Grilled Chicken Salad:

Ingredients:

- 2 boneless, skinless chicken breasts
- Salt and black pepper to taste
- 1 teaspoon paprika
- 1 teaspoon garlic powder
- 1 teaspoon dried oregano
- 2 tablespoons olive oil (for marinating and grilling)
- 6 cups mixed salad greens (lettuce, spinach, arugula)
- 1 cup cherry tomatoes, halved
- 1 cucumber, sliced
- 1/2 red onion, thinly sliced
- 1/4 cup feta cheese, crumbled

- 1/4 cup Kalamata olives, pitted
- Balsamic vinaigrette dressing

Instructions:

1. Preheat the grill or grill pan over medium-high heat.
2. Season chicken breasts with salt, black pepper, paprika, garlic powder, and dried oregano.
3. Drizzle olive oil over the seasoned chicken breasts and rub to coat evenly.
4. Grill the chicken for about 6-8 minutes per side or until fully cooked. Ensure the internal temperature reaches 165°F (74°C).
5. Allow the grilled chicken to rest for a few minutes before slicing it into thin strips.
6. In a large bowl, combine mixed salad greens, cherry tomatoes, cucumber, red onion, feta cheese, and Kalamata olives.
7. Add the sliced grilled chicken on top of the salad.
8. Drizzle balsamic vinaigrette dressing over the salad, tossing gently to coat all ingredients.
9. Serve immediately, and enjoy your flavorful and satisfying Grilled Chicken Salad!

Quinoa and Black Bean Bowl:

Ingredients:

- 1 cup quinoa, rinsed
- 2 cups vegetable broth or water
- 1 can (15 oz) black beans, drained and rinsed
- 1 cup corn kernels (fresh, frozen, or canned)
- 1 red bell pepper, diced
- 1 avocado, sliced
- 1/4 cup chopped fresh cilantro
- Juice of 1 lime
- 1 teaspoon ground cumin
- 1 teaspoon chili powder

- Salt and pepper to taste
- Optional toppings: salsa, Greek yogurt, shredded cheese

Instructions:

1. In a medium saucepan, combine quinoa and vegetable broth (or water). Bring to a boil, then reduce heat, cover, and simmer for about 15 minutes or until quinoa is cooked and liquid is absorbed.
2. While quinoa is cooking, in a separate pan, heat black beans, corn, and diced red bell pepper over medium heat. Add ground cumin, chili powder, salt, and pepper. Cook until vegetables are tender and the mixture is heated through.
3. Once quinoa is cooked, fluff it with a fork and transfer it to a serving bowl.
4. Spoon the black bean and vegetable mixture over the quinoa.
5. Squeeze lime juice over the bowl and toss gently to combine.
6. Top with sliced avocado and chopped cilantro.
7. If desired, add optional toppings such as salsa, Greek yogurt, or shredded cheese.
8. Serve warm and enjoy your nutritious and flavorful Quinoa and Black Bean Bowl!

Salmon and Vegetable Stir-Fry:

Ingredients:

- 1 lb salmon filets, cut into bite-sized pieces
- 2 tablespoons soy sauce
- 1 tablespoon oyster sauce
- 1 tablespoon hoisin sauce
- 1 tablespoon sesame oil
- 2 tablespoons vegetable oil
- 3 cups mixed vegetables (broccoli florets, bell peppers, snap peas, carrots), chopped
- 3 cloves garlic, minced
- 1 tablespoon ginger, grated
- 2 green onions, sliced

- Sesame seeds for garnish (optional)
- Cooked rice or noodles for serving

Instructions:

1. In a bowl, mix soy sauce, oyster sauce, and hoisin sauce to create the stir-fry sauce.
2. Season salmon pieces with a pinch of salt and pepper.
3. In a large skillet or wok, heat vegetable oil over medium-high heat.
4. Add salmon to the skillet and cook for 2-3 minutes on each side until browned and cooked through. Remove salmon from the skillet and set aside.
5. In the same skillet, add sesame oil. Stir in garlic and ginger, cooking for about 30 seconds until fragrant.
6. Add mixed vegetables to the skillet and stir-fry for 3-4 minutes until they are slightly tender but still crisp.
7. Return the cooked salmon to the skillet with the vegetables.
8. Pour the stir-fry sauce over the salmon and vegetables. Toss everything together until well coated and heated through.
9. Stir in sliced green onions and cook for an additional 1-2 minutes.
10. Serve the Salmon and Vegetable Stir-Fry over cooked rice or noodles.
11. Garnish with sesame seeds if desired.

Turkey and Hummus Wrap:

Ingredients:

- 1 large whole-grain or spinach tortilla
- 4 slices of deli turkey
- 2 tablespoons hummus
- 1/2 cup mixed salad greens
- 1/4 cup cherry tomatoes, halved
- 1/4 cucumber, sliced
- 1/4 red onion, thinly sliced

- 1 tablespoon feta cheese, crumbled (optional)
- Salt and black pepper to taste

Instructions:

1. Lay the tortilla flat on a clean surface.
2. Spread hummus evenly over the entire surface of the tortilla.
3. Place the turkey slices on one half of the tortilla, leaving space at the edges.
4. In a bowl, toss together mixed salad greens, cherry tomatoes, cucumber, and red onion.
5. Pile the salad mixture onto the same half of the tortilla as the turkey.
6. If using, sprinkle feta cheese over the salad.
7. Season with salt and black pepper to taste.
8. Starting from the side with the turkey, tightly roll the tortilla into a wrap, enclosing the filling.
9. Slice the wrap in half at a slight diagonal for easier handling.
10. Secure each half with toothpicks if needed.

Vegetarian Chickpea Salad:

Ingredients:

- 2 cans (15 oz each) chickpeas, drained and rinsed
- 1 cup cherry tomatoes, halved
- 1 cucumber, diced
- 1/2 red onion, finely chopped
- 1 bell pepper (any color), diced
- 1/4 cup Kalamata olives, pitted and sliced
- 1/4 cup feta cheese, crumbled
- 1/4 cup fresh parsley, chopped
- 3 tablespoons extra virgin olive oil
- 2 tablespoons red wine vinegar
- 1 teaspoon Dijon mustard

- 1 clove garlic, minced
- Salt and black pepper to taste

Instructions:

1. In a large mixing bowl, combine chickpeas, cherry tomatoes, cucumber, red onion, bell pepper, olives, feta cheese, and fresh parsley.
2. In a small bowl, whisk together olive oil, red wine vinegar, Dijon mustard, minced garlic, salt, and black pepper to create the dressing.
3. Pour the dressing over the chickpea mixture and toss gently until well combined.
4. Taste and adjust salt and pepper as needed.
5. Let the salad marinate in the refrigerator for at least 30 minutes to allow the flavors to meld.
6. Before serving, give the salad a final toss.
7. Serve chilled and enjoy your refreshing Vegetarian Chickpea Salad!

Quinoa Stuffed Bell Peppers:

Ingredients:

- 4 large bell peppers, halved and seeds removed
- 1 cup quinoa, rinsed
- 2 cups vegetable broth or water
- 1 tablespoon olive oil
- 1 onion, finely chopped
- 2 cloves garlic, minced
- 1 zucchini, diced
- 1 carrot, grated
- 1 can (15 oz) black beans, drained and rinsed
- 1 cup corn kernels (fresh, frozen, or canned)
- 1 teaspoon ground cumin
- 1 teaspoon chili powder
- Salt and black pepper to taste

- 1 cup tomato sauce or salsa
- 1 cup shredded cheese (cheddar, Monterey Jack, or your choice)
- Fresh cilantro or parsley for garnish (optional)

Instructions:

1. Preheat the oven to 375°F (190°C).
2. In a saucepan, combine quinoa and vegetable broth (or water). Bring to a boil, then reduce heat, cover, and simmer for about 15 minutes or until quinoa is cooked and liquid is absorbed.
3. While quinoa is cooking, heat olive oil in a skillet over medium heat.
4. Sauté onion and garlic until softened.
5. Add diced zucchini and grated carrot to the skillet. Cook until vegetables are tender.
6. Stir in black beans, corn, ground cumin, chili powder, salt, and black pepper. Cook for an additional 2-3 minutes.
7. In a large mixing bowl, combine the cooked quinoa with the sautéed vegetable mixture.
8. Place the halved bell peppers in a baking dish.
9. Spoon the quinoa and vegetable mixture into each bell pepper half.
10. Pour tomato sauce or salsa over the stuffed peppers.
11. Sprinkle shredded cheese on top of each stuffed pepper.
12. Cover the baking dish with aluminum foil and bake for 25-30 minutes, or until peppers are tender.
13. Remove the foil and bake for an additional 5-10 minutes until the cheese is melted and bubbly.
14. Garnish with fresh cilantro or parsley if desired.

Shrimp and Avocado Lettuce Wraps:

Ingredients:

- 1 pound large shrimp, peeled and deveined

- 1 tablespoon olive oil
- 1 teaspoon smoked paprika
- 1 teaspoon garlic powder
- Salt and black pepper to taste
- Juice of 1 lime
- 1 avocado, diced
- 1/2 cup cherry tomatoes, halved
- 1/4 cup red onion, finely chopped
- 1/4 cup fresh cilantro, chopped
- Butter lettuce leaves for wrapping

Instructions:

1. In a bowl, toss shrimp with olive oil, smoked paprika, garlic powder, salt, and black pepper.
2. Heat a skillet over medium-high heat. Add the seasoned shrimp and cook for 2-3 minutes per side or until they turn pink and opaque.
3. Squeeze lime juice over the cooked shrimp and toss to coat. Remove from heat.
4. In a separate bowl, combine diced avocado, cherry tomatoes, red onion, and fresh cilantro.
5. Place a spoonful of the avocado mixture onto each butter lettuce leaf.
6. Top with a few cooked shrimp on each lettuce leaf.
7. Optionally, drizzle extra lime juice over the wraps for added freshness.
8. Serve your Shrimp and Avocado Lettuce Wraps immediately.

Mushroom and Spinach Frittata:

Ingredients:

- 8 large eggs
- 1/4 cup milk
- Salt and black pepper to taste
- 1 tablespoon olive oil

- 1 onion, diced
- 8 oz mushrooms, sliced
- 2 cups fresh spinach, chopped
- 1/2 cup feta cheese, crumbled
- Fresh herbs (such as parsley or chives) for garnish

Instructions:

1. Preheat the oven to 350°F (175°C).
2. In a bowl, whisk together eggs, milk, salt, and black pepper until well combined.
3. Heat olive oil in an oven-safe skillet over medium heat.
4. Add diced onion to the skillet and sauté until translucent.
5. Add sliced mushrooms and cook until they release their moisture and become golden brown.
6. Stir in chopped spinach and cook until wilted.
7. Spread the vegetable mixture evenly in the skillet.
8. Pour the whisked egg mixture over the vegetables.
9. Sprinkle crumbled feta cheese over the top.
10. Cook on the stovetop for 2-3 minutes until the edges begin to set.
11. Transfer the skillet to the preheated oven and bake for 15-20 minutes or until the frittata is set in the middle and the top is lightly golden.
12. Carefully remove from the oven and let it cool for a few minutes.
13. Garnish with fresh herbs.
14. Slice and serve your Mushroom and Spinach Frittata warm.

Lentil Soup:

Ingredients:

- 1 cup dried lentils, rinsed and drained
- 1 onion, finely chopped
- 2 carrots, diced
- 2 celery stalks, diced

- 3 cloves garlic, minced
- 1 can (14 oz) diced tomatoes
- 6 cups vegetable or chicken broth
- 1 teaspoon ground cumin
- 1 teaspoon ground coriander
- 1/2 teaspoon smoked paprika
- 1 bay leaf
- Salt and black pepper to taste
- 2 tablespoons olive oil
- Juice of 1 lemon
- Fresh parsley for garnish (optional)

Instructions:

1. In a large pot, heat olive oil over medium heat.
2. Add chopped onion, carrots, and celery. Sauté until the vegetables are softened.
3. Add minced garlic and cook for an additional 1-2 minutes until fragrant.
4. Stir in ground cumin, ground coriander, and smoked paprika.
5. Add dried lentils, diced tomatoes (with their juice), bay leaf, and vegetable or chicken broth to the pot.
6. Season with salt and black pepper to taste.
7. Bring the soup to a boil, then reduce the heat to low, cover, and simmer for about 25-30 minutes or until the lentils are tender.
8. Discard the bay leaf.
9. Stir in lemon juice for a bright, fresh flavor.
10. Taste and adjust the seasoning if necessary.
11. If desired, garnish with fresh parsley before serving.

Sweet Potato and Chickpea Buddha Bowl:

Ingredients:

- 1 large sweet potato, peeled and cubed

- 1 can (15 oz) chickpeas, drained and rinsed
- 1 tablespoon olive oil
- 1 teaspoon ground cumin
- 1 teaspoon paprika
- Salt and pepper to taste
- 2 cups cooked quinoa or brown rice
- 2 cups kale, stems removed and chopped
- 1 avocado, sliced
- 1/4 cup hummus
- Sesame seeds for garnish

For the Tahini Dressing:

- 3 tablespoons tahini
- 2 tablespoons lemon juice
- 1 tablespoon maple syrup
- 2 tablespoons water
- Salt and pepper to taste

Instructions:

1. Preheat the oven to 400°F (200°C).
2. In a bowl, toss the sweet potato cubes and chickpeas with olive oil, cumin, paprika, salt, and pepper until evenly coated.
3. Spread the sweet potato and chickpea mixture on a baking sheet in a single layer. Roast in the preheated oven for 25-30 minutes or until the sweet potatoes are tender and chickpeas are crispy, stirring halfway through.
4. While the vegetables are roasting, prepare the tahini dressing by whisking together tahini, lemon juice, maple syrup, water, salt, and pepper. Adjust the consistency with more water if needed.
5. In a large bowl, assemble the Buddha bowls by dividing cooked quinoa or brown rice among serving bowls.

6. Top with roasted sweet potatoes and chickpeas, chopped kale, avocado slices, and a dollop of hummus.

7. Drizzle the tahini dressing over the bowls and sprinkle with sesame seeds.

8. Serve immediately and enjoy your nutritious and flavorful Sweet Potato and Chickpea Buddha Bowl!

Caprese Salad with Grilled Chicken:

Ingredients:

- 2 boneless, skinless chicken breasts
- Salt and pepper to taste
- 1 tablespoon olive oil
- 2 teaspoons Italian seasoning
- 1 teaspoon garlic powder

For the Salad:

- 4 large tomatoes, sliced
- 1 pound fresh mozzarella cheese, sliced
- Fresh basil leaves
- Balsamic glaze for drizzling
- Salt and pepper to taste

Instructions:

1. Preheat the grill to medium-high heat.

2. Season the chicken breasts with salt, pepper, Italian seasoning, and garlic powder. Drizzle with olive oil and rub the seasonings into the chicken.

3. Grill the chicken breasts for about 6-8 minutes per side or until fully cooked and no longer pink in the center. The internal temperature should reach 165°F (74°C).

4. While the chicken is grilling, arrange the tomato and mozzarella slices on a serving platter, alternating them.

5. Once the chicken is cooked, let it rest for a few minutes before slicing it into thin strips.

6. Place the grilled chicken strips on top of the tomato and mozzarella slices.

7. Tuck fresh basil leaves between the chicken, tomatoes, and mozzarella.

8. Drizzle the entire salad with balsamic glaze and season with salt and pepper to taste.

9. Serve immediately, allowing the flavors to meld together, and enjoy this delicious Caprese Salad with Grilled Chicken!

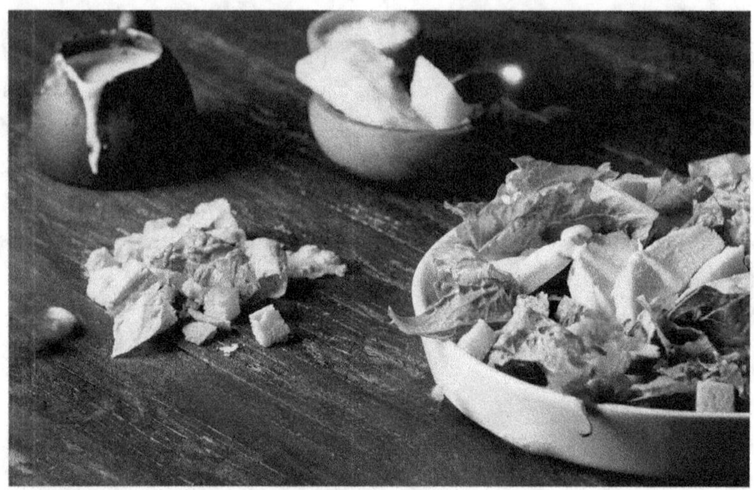

Baked Lemon Herb Chicken:

Ingredients:

- 4 boneless, skinless chicken breasts
- 2 tablespoons olive oil
- 3 tablespoons lemon juice
- Zest of one lemon
- 2 cloves garlic, minced
- 1 teaspoon dried oregano
- 1 teaspoon dried thyme
- 1 teaspoon dried rosemary
- Salt and pepper to taste
- Lemon slices for garnish (optional)
- Fresh parsley for garnish (optional)

Instructions:

1. Preheat the oven to 400°F (200°C).

2. In a small bowl, whisk together olive oil, lemon juice, lemon zest, minced garlic, dried oregano, dried thyme, dried rosemary, salt, and pepper.

3. Place the chicken breasts in a resealable plastic bag or shallow dish. Pour the lemon herb marinade over the chicken, ensuring it's well-coated. Marinate in the refrigerator for at least 30 minutes to let the flavors infuse.

4. Remove the chicken from the refrigerator and let it come to room temperature for about 10-15 minutes.

5. Place the marinated chicken breasts in a baking dish.

6. Bake in the preheated oven for 20-25 minutes or until the chicken reaches an internal temperature of 165°F (74°C), and the juices run clear.

7. If desired, garnish the baked lemon herb chicken with lemon slices and fresh parsley before serving.

8. Serve the deliciously baked lemon herb chicken with your favorite sides and enjoy!

Vegetable Stir-Fry with Tofu:

Ingredients:

- 1 block extra-firm tofu, pressed and cubed
- 2 tablespoons soy sauce
- 1 tablespoon sesame oil
- 1 tablespoon cornstarch
- 2 tablespoons vegetable oil, divided
- 2 cups broccoli florets
- 1 red bell pepper, sliced
- 1 yellow bell pepper, sliced
- 1 carrot, julienned
- 1 zucchini, sliced

- 3 green onions, sliced
- 2 cloves garlic, minced
- 1 teaspoon ginger, minced
- 1/4 cup soy sauce (additional for stir-frying)
- 2 tablespoons hoisin sauce
- 1 tablespoon rice vinegar
- 1 tablespoon brown sugar
- Sesame seeds for garnish (optional)
- Cooked rice or noodles for serving

Instructions:

1. In a bowl, combine cubed tofu with soy sauce, sesame oil, and cornstarch. Gently toss to coat the tofu evenly. Let it marinate for at least 15 minutes.
2. Heat 1 tablespoon of vegetable oil in a large wok or skillet over medium-high heat. Add the marinated tofu and cook until golden brown on all sides. Remove tofu from the wok and set aside.
3. In the same wok, add the remaining tablespoon of vegetable oil. Add garlic and ginger, sauté for about 30 seconds until fragrant.
4. Add broccoli, bell peppers, carrot, and zucchini to the wok. Stir-fry for 4-5 minutes or until the vegetables are tender-crisp.
5. In a small bowl, whisk together soy sauce, hoisin sauce, rice vinegar, and brown sugar. Pour the sauce over the vegetables in the wok.
6. Add the cooked tofu back into the wok and toss everything together until well coated in the sauce.
7. Stir in sliced green onions and cook for an additional 1-2 minutes.
8. Serve the vegetable stir-fry with tofu over cooked rice or noodles. Garnish with sesame seeds if desired.

Salmon with Quinoa and Roasted Vegetables:

Ingredients:

- 4 salmon fillets
- 1 cup quinoa, rinsed
- 2 cups cherry tomatoes, halved
- 1 red bell pepper, sliced
- 1 zucchini, sliced
- 1 red onion, sliced
- 3 tablespoons olive oil, divided
- 2 cloves garlic, minced
- 1 teaspoon dried thyme
- 1 teaspoon dried rosemary
- Salt and pepper to taste
- Lemon wedges for serving
- Fresh parsley for garnish (optional)

Instructions:

1. Preheat the oven to 400°F (200°C).
2. In a saucepan, combine quinoa with 2 cups of water. Bring to a boil, then reduce heat to low, cover, and simmer for 15 minutes or until the quinoa is cooked and water is absorbed. Fluff with a fork.
3. Place the salmon fillets on a baking sheet lined with parchment paper. Drizzle with 1 tablespoon of olive oil and season with salt and pepper.
4. In a large bowl, toss the cherry tomatoes, red bell pepper, zucchini, and red onion with 2 tablespoons of olive oil, minced garlic, dried thyme, dried rosemary, salt, and pepper.
5. Spread the vegetable mixture around the salmon fillets on the baking sheet.
6. Roast in the preheated oven for 15-20 minutes or until the salmon is cooked through and flakes easily with a fork, and the vegetables are tender.
7. While the salmon and vegetables are roasting, divide the cooked quinoa among serving plates.

8. Place a roasted salmon fillet on each bed of quinoa and spoon the roasted vegetables over the top.

9. Garnish with fresh parsley if desired and serve with lemon wedges on the side.

Turkey and Vegetable Skewers:

Ingredients:

- 1.5 lbs (700g) turkey breast, cut into cubes
- 1 red bell pepper, cut into chunks
- 1 yellow bell pepper, cut into chunks
- 1 zucchini, sliced
- 1 red onion, cut into chunks
- 1/4 cup olive oil
- 2 tablespoons soy sauce
- 2 tablespoons honey
- 2 cloves garlic, minced
- 1 teaspoon dried oregano
- 1 teaspoon smoked paprika
- Salt and pepper to taste
- Wooden or metal skewers

Instructions:

1. If using wooden skewers, soak them in water for at least 30 minutes to prevent burning during cooking.

2. In a bowl, whisk together olive oil, soy sauce, honey, minced garlic, dried oregano, smoked paprika, salt, and pepper to create the marinade.

3. Thread turkey cubes, bell pepper chunks, zucchini slices, and red onion chunks onto the skewers, alternating the ingredients.

4. Place the assembled skewers in a shallow dish and brush the marinade over them, ensuring even coating. Let them marinate for at least 30 minutes.

5. Preheat the grill or grill pan to medium-high heat.

6. Grill the turkey and vegetable skewers for about 10-12 minutes, turning occasionally, until the turkey is cooked through and vegetables are tender.

7. During grilling, baste the skewers with the remaining marinade for added flavor.

8. Once cooked, transfer the skewers to a serving platter.

Mushroom and Spinach Stuffed Chicken Breast:

Ingredients:

- 4 boneless, skinless chicken breasts
- Salt and pepper to taste
- 2 tablespoons olive oil, divided
- 2 cups mushrooms, finely chopped
- 2 cups fresh spinach, chopped
- 2 cloves garlic, minced
- 1/2 cup shredded mozzarella cheese
- 1/4 cup grated Parmesan cheese
- 1 teaspoon dried thyme
- 1 teaspoon dried rosemary
- 1/2 cup chicken broth
- Toothpicks or kitchen twine

Instructions:

1. Preheat the oven to 375°F (190°C).

2. Season each chicken breast with salt and pepper. Use a sharp knife to make a horizontal slit along the side of each breast, creating a pocket for stuffing. Be careful not to cut all the way through.

3. In a skillet, heat 1 tablespoon of olive oil over medium heat. Add chopped mushrooms and sauté until they release their moisture and become golden brown. Add minced garlic and cook for an additional minute.

4. Add chopped spinach to the skillet and cook until wilted. Remove the skillet from heat and let the mixture cool slightly.

5. Stir in mozzarella cheese, Parmesan cheese, dried thyme, and dried rosemary into the mushroom and spinach mixture.

6. Stuff each chicken breast with the mushroom and spinach mixture, using toothpicks or kitchen twine to secure the openings.

7. In the same skillet, heat the remaining tablespoon of olive oil. Place the stuffed chicken breasts in the skillet and sear on each side until golden brown.

8. Pour chicken broth into the skillet, and then transfer the skillet to the preheated oven.

9. Bake for 20-25 minutes or until the chicken is cooked through (reaching an internal temperature of 165°F or 74°C) and the cheese is melted and bubbly.

10. Remove toothpicks or twine before serving.

Cauliflower Crust Pizza:

Ingredients:

For the Cauliflower Crust:

- 1 medium-sized cauliflower head, riced (about 4 cups)
- 1/2 cup mozzarella cheese, shredded
- 1/4 cup Parmesan cheese, grated
- 1 teaspoon dried oregano
- 1 teaspoon dried basil
- 1/2 teaspoon garlic powder
- 1/4 teaspoon salt
- 1/4 teaspoon black pepper
- 2 large eggs

For Topping:

- 1/2 cup pizza sauce
- 1 to 1.5 cups shredded mozzarella cheese
- Your favorite pizza toppings (e.g., cherry tomatoes, bell peppers, olives, basil)

Instructions:

1. Preheat the oven to 400°F (200°C). Place a pizza stone or a baking sheet in the oven to heat.
2. Rice the cauliflower by either using a food processor or grating it with a box grater. Microwave the riced cauliflower for 5-6 minutes or until tender. Allow it to cool.
3. Place the cooled cauliflower in a clean kitchen towel or cheesecloth, and wring out as much moisture as possible. This step is crucial for a crisp crust.
4. In a bowl, combine the cauliflower with shredded mozzarella, grated Parmesan, dried oregano, dried basil, garlic powder, salt, and black pepper.
5. Add the eggs to the cauliflower mixture and mix until a dough forms.
6. Place parchment paper on a pizza peel or another baking sheet. Spread the cauliflower dough onto the parchment paper, shaping it into a round pizza crust.
7. Slide the parchment paper onto the preheated pizza stone or baking sheet in the oven. Bake for 20-25 minutes or until the crust is golden brown and firm.
8. Remove the crust from the oven and spread pizza sauce, shredded mozzarella, and your favorite toppings.
9. Place the pizza back in the oven and bake for an additional 10-15 minutes or until the cheese is melted and bubbly.
10. Remove the cauliflower crust pizza from the oven, let it cool for a few minutes, slice, and enjoy your low-carb and gluten-free pizza!

Shrimp and Zucchini Noodles:

Ingredients:

- 1 pound (450g) large shrimp, peeled and deveined
- 3 medium zucchinis, spiralized into noodles
- 3 tablespoons olive oil, divided
- 4 cloves garlic, minced
- 1 teaspoon red pepper flakes (optional)
- Salt and black pepper to taste

- Juice of 1 lemon
- 2 tablespoons chopped fresh parsley
- Grated Parmesan cheese for garnish (optional)

Instructions:

1. In a large skillet, heat 2 tablespoons of olive oil over medium-high heat.
2. Add shrimp to the skillet and cook for 2-3 minutes per side or until they turn pink and opaque. Season with salt and black pepper. Once cooked, remove the shrimp from the skillet and set aside.
3. In the same skillet, add the remaining tablespoon of olive oil. Add minced garlic and red pepper flakes (if using) and sauté for about 1 minute until fragrant.
4. Add spiralized zucchini noodles to the skillet. Toss the noodles with the garlic and oil, cooking for 2-3 minutes until just tender. Be careful not to overcook; zucchini noodles should be al dente.
5. Return the cooked shrimp to the skillet, tossing them with the zucchini noodles to combine.
6. Drizzle lemon juice over the mixture, stirring to incorporate the flavors. Adjust salt and pepper to taste.
7. Sprinkle chopped fresh parsley over the shrimp and zucchini noodles.
8. Serve the dish hot, garnished with grated Parmesan cheese if desired.

Eggplant Parmesan:

Ingredients:

- 2 large eggplants, sliced into 1/2-inch rounds
- Salt for sweating eggplant
- 2 cups all-purpose flour, for dredging
- 4 large eggs
- 2 tablespoons water
- 2 cups breadcrumbs
- 1 cup grated Parmesan cheese

- 2 cups marinara sauce
- 2 cups shredded mozzarella cheese
- 1/4 cup fresh basil leaves, chopped
- Olive oil for frying
- Salt and pepper to taste

Instructions:

1. Preheat the oven to 375°F (190°C).

2. Place eggplant slices on a baking sheet, sprinkle with salt, and let them sit for 30 minutes. This helps remove excess moisture and bitterness. After 30 minutes, pat the eggplant slices dry with paper towels.

3. Set up a dredging station: Place flour in one bowl, whisk eggs with water in another bowl, and combine breadcrumbs with grated Parmesan in a third bowl.

4. Heat olive oil in a large skillet over medium-high heat.

5. Dredge each eggplant slice in flour, dip into the egg mixture, and coat with the breadcrumb-Parmesan mixture.

6. Fry the coated eggplant slices in batches until golden brown on both sides. Place the fried slices on paper towels to absorb excess oil.

7. In a baking dish, spread a thin layer of marinara sauce. Arrange a layer of fried eggplant slices on top.

8. Sprinkle shredded mozzarella cheese and chopped fresh basil over the eggplant layer. Repeat the process, creating layers until all ingredients are used, finishing with a layer of mozzarella on top.

9. Bake in the preheated oven for 25-30 minutes or until the cheese is melted and bubbly, and the edges are golden brown.

10. Allow the Eggplant Parmesan to cool for a few minutes before slicing and serving.

11. Garnish with additional fresh basil and Parmesan if desired.

12. Enjoy your homemade Eggplant Parmesan served with a side of pasta or a green salad!

Quinoa and Black Bean Stuffed Peppers:

Ingredients:

- 4 large bell peppers, halved and seeds removed
- 1 cup quinoa, rinsed
- 2 cups vegetable broth or water
- 1 can (15 oz) black beans, drained and rinsed
- 1 cup corn kernels (fresh or frozen)
- 1 cup diced tomatoes
- 1 cup diced red onion
- 2 cloves garlic, minced
- 1 teaspoon ground cumin
- 1 teaspoon chili powder
- Salt and pepper to taste
- 1 cup shredded Mexican blend cheese
- Fresh cilantro for garnish (optional)
- Lime wedges for serving

Instructions:

1. Preheat the oven to 375°F (190°C).
2. In a medium saucepan, combine quinoa and vegetable broth (or water). Bring to a boil, then reduce heat to low, cover, and simmer for 15-20 minutes or until the quinoa is cooked and the liquid is absorbed.
3. In a large bowl, mix together cooked quinoa, black beans, corn, diced tomatoes, red onion, minced garlic, ground cumin, chili powder, salt, and pepper.
4. Place the halved bell peppers in a baking dish, cut side up.
5. Stuff each pepper half with the quinoa and black bean mixture, pressing it down gently.
6. Sprinkle shredded cheese over the top of each stuffed pepper.
7. Cover the baking dish with foil and bake in the preheated oven for 25-30 minutes or until the peppers are tender.

8. Remove the foil and bake for an additional 5-10 minutes until the cheese is melted and bubbly.

9. Garnish the Quinoa and Black Bean Stuffed Peppers with fresh cilantro if desired.

10. Serve hot with lime wedges on the side for squeezing over the peppers.

Chickpea Curry:

Ingredients:

- 2 cans (15 oz each) chickpeas, drained and rinsed
- 1 large onion, finely chopped
- 3 cloves garlic, minced
- 1 tablespoon ginger, grated
- 1 can (14 oz) diced tomatoes
- 1 can (14 oz) coconut milk
- 2 tablespoons curry powder
- 1 teaspoon ground cumin
- 1 teaspoon ground coriander
- 1/2 teaspoon turmeric
- 1/2 teaspoon cayenne pepper (adjust to taste)
- Salt and pepper to taste
- 2 tablespoons vegetable oil
- Fresh cilantro for garnish (optional)
- Cooked rice or naan for serving

Instructions:

1. In a large skillet or pot, heat vegetable oil over medium heat.

2. Add chopped onions and sauté until translucent.

3. Add minced garlic and grated ginger, sauté for an additional 1-2 minutes until fragrant.

4. Stir in curry powder, ground cumin, ground coriander, turmeric, cayenne pepper, salt, and pepper. Cook the spices for 1-2 minutes to release their flavors.

5. Pour in the diced tomatoes (with their juice) and coconut milk. Stir to combine.

6. Add drained chickpeas to the pot, stirring well to coat them in the curry sauce.

7. Bring the mixture to a simmer, then reduce the heat to low, cover, and let it simmer for 15-20 minutes, allowing the flavors to meld together.

8. Taste and adjust seasoning if necessary.

9. If you prefer a thicker curry, you can mash some of the chickpeas with the back of a spoon or use an immersion blender to partially blend the mixture.

10. Serve the chickpea curry over cooked rice or with naan.

11. Garnish with fresh cilantro if desired.

Grilled Vegetable and Chicken Kabobs:

Ingredients:

- 1.5 lbs (700g) boneless, skinless chicken breasts, cut into bite-sized pieces
- 1 zucchini, sliced
- 1 red bell pepper, cut into chunks
- 1 yellow bell pepper, cut into chunks
- 1 red onion, cut into chunks
- 8-10 cherry tomatoes
- 1/4 cup olive oil
- 2 tablespoons balsamic vinegar
- 2 cloves garlic, minced
- 1 teaspoon dried oregano
- 1 teaspoon dried thyme
- Salt and pepper to taste
- Wooden or metal skewers

Instructions:

1. If using wooden skewers, soak them in water for at least 30 minutes to prevent burning during grilling.

2. In a bowl, combine olive oil, balsamic vinegar, minced garlic, dried oregano, dried thyme, salt, and pepper to create the marinade.

3. Place chicken pieces in the marinade, ensuring they are well-coated. Allow them to marinate for at least 30 minutes.

4. Preheat the grill to medium-high heat.

5. Thread marinated chicken, zucchini slices, bell pepper chunks, red onion chunks, and cherry tomatoes onto the skewers, alternating the ingredients.

6. Brush the assembled kabobs with any remaining marinade.

7. Grill the kabobs for about 12-15 minutes, turning occasionally, until the chicken is cooked through, and the vegetables are tender and slightly charred.

8. During grilling, baste the kabobs with additional marinade for added flavor.

9. Once cooked, remove the kabobs from the grill and let them rest for a few minutes.

10. Serve the Grilled Vegetable and Chicken Kabobs hot, and enjoy this flavorful and colorful dish!

CHAPTER 6: SNACKS AND APPETIZERS

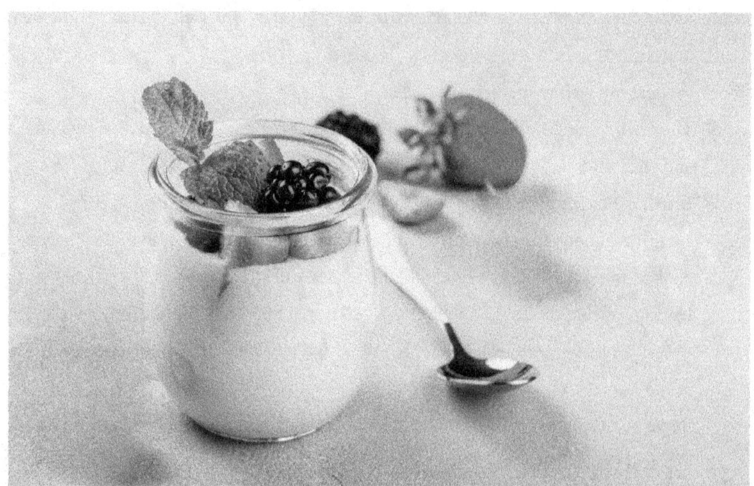

Greek Yogurt with Berries:

Ingredients:

- 1 cup Greek yogurt (plain or vanilla)
- 1 cup mixed berries (strawberries, blueberries, raspberries, blackberries)
- 1-2 tablespoons honey or maple syrup (optional)
- 1/4 cup granola (optional)
- Fresh mint leaves for garnish (optional)

Instructions:

1. Spoon Greek yogurt into a serving bowl.
2. Wash and prepare the mixed berries. If using strawberries, hull and slice them.
3. Arrange the mixed berries on top of the Greek yogurt.
4. If desired, drizzle honey or maple syrup over the yogurt and berries for a touch of sweetness.

5. Optionally, sprinkle granola over the top for added crunch and texture.

6. Garnish with fresh mint leaves for a burst of freshness.

7. Mix the ingredients gently just before eating to combine the flavors.

8. Serve immediately and enjoy this simple and nutritious Greek Yogurt with Berries as a refreshing snack or breakfast!

Almond Butter and Banana Slices:

Ingredients:

- 2 medium-sized bananas, peeled and sliced
- 1/4 cup almond butter
- Optional toppings: Chia seeds, shredded coconut, chopped nuts, drizzle of honey

Instructions:

1. Peel and slice the bananas into rounds.

2. Spread a thin layer of almond butter onto each banana slice.

3. Arrange the almond butter-coated banana slices on a serving plate.

4. Optional: Drizzle a small amount of honey over the banana slices for added sweetness.

5. Sprinkle chia seeds, shredded coconut, or chopped nuts on top for extra texture and flavor.

6. Serve immediately and enjoy these Almond Butter and Banana Slices as a quick and delicious snack or a healthy breakfast option!

Hummus and Veggie Sticks:

Ingredients:

- 1 cup hummus (store-bought or homemade)
- Assorted veggies for dipping (carrot sticks, cucumber slices, bell pepper strips, cherry tomatoes, etc.)

Instructions:

1. If making homemade hummus, blend chickpeas, tahini, lemon juice, garlic, olive oil, and salt in a food processor until smooth. Adjust the consistency with water if needed.
2. Wash, peel, and cut assorted veggies into sticks or slices suitable for dipping.
3. Arrange the veggie sticks on a serving platter.
4. Place a bowl of hummus in the center of the veggie arrangement.
5. Serve immediately and enjoy Hummus and Veggie Sticks as a nutritious and satisfying snack or appetizer!
6. Optionally, you can sprinkle a bit of paprika or drizzle olive oil over the hummus for extra flavor.

Mixed Nuts:

Ingredients:

- 2 cups mixed nuts (almonds, walnuts, cashews, pecans, etc.)
- 1 tablespoon olive oil or melted butter
- 1 tablespoon honey or maple syrup
- 1 teaspoon ground cinnamon (optional)
- 1/2 teaspoon salt (adjust to taste)

Instructions:

1. Preheat the oven to 325°F (163°C).
2. In a bowl, combine mixed nuts with olive oil or melted butter, ensuring they are well-coated.
3. Drizzle honey or maple syrup over the nuts and toss to evenly distribute the sweetness.
4. If desired, sprinkle ground cinnamon over the nuts for added flavor.
5. Spread the coated nuts in a single layer on a baking sheet lined with parchment paper.
6. Bake in the preheated oven for 15-20 minutes, stirring halfway through, until the nuts are golden and fragrant.

7. Remove the mixed nuts from the oven and immediately sprinkle with salt, tossing them while still warm.

8. Let the mixed nuts cool completely before storing in an airtight container.

Cheese and Whole Grain Crackers:

Ingredients:

- Assorted whole grain crackers
- Variety of cheeses (cheddar, brie, gouda, etc.), sliced or cubed
- Grapes or apple slices (optional, for serving)

Instructions:

1. Arrange the whole grain crackers on a serving platter or plate.
2. Place slices or cubes of different cheeses alongside the crackers.
3. Optionally, add grapes or apple slices to the platter for a sweet contrast.
4. Serve the Cheese and Whole Grain Crackers as a delightful snack or appetizer for gatherings.
5. Enjoy the combination of wholesome crackers and flavorful cheeses, creating a balanced and satisfying snack!

Apple Slices with Peanut Butter:

Ingredients:

- 2 apples (any variety), cored and sliced
- 1/2 cup peanut butter (smooth or crunchy)
- Optional toppings: Honey, chia seeds, granola, shredded coconut

Instructions:

1. Core and slice the apples into thin rounds or wedges.
2. Place peanut butter in a small bowl for dipping.
3. Optionally, drizzle honey over the peanut butter for added sweetness.
4. Arrange the apple slices on a serving plate.
5. Dip each apple slice into the peanut butter or spread peanut butter on each slice.

6. Optional: Sprinkle chia seeds, granola, or shredded coconut on top of the peanut butter.

7. Serve immediately and enjoy Apple Slices with Peanut Butter as a wholesome and satisfying snack!

8. Experiment with different toppings or nut butter variations for added variety.

Hard-Boiled Eggs:

Ingredients:

- Eggs (as many as desired)

Instructions:

1. Place the eggs in a single layer in a saucepan or pot.

2. Add enough water to the pot to cover the eggs by about an inch.

3. Place the pot on the stove over medium-high heat.

4. Once the water reaches a boil, reduce the heat to a simmer.

5. Simmer the eggs for 9-12 minutes, depending on your desired yolk consistency:
   - 9 minutes for a creamy yolk
   - 10-12 minutes for a firmer yolk

6. While the eggs are simmering, prepare a bowl of ice water.

7. Once the eggs are done, immediately transfer them to the ice water using a slotted spoon. This helps stop the cooking process and makes peeling easier.

8. Let the eggs sit in the ice water for at least 5 minutes.

9. Gently tap each egg on a hard surface to crack the shell, then peel the shell away.

10. Rinse the peeled eggs under cold water to remove any remaining shell pieces.

11. Pat the eggs dry with a paper towel.

12. Enjoy your perfectly cooked Hard-Boiled Eggs as a snack, salad topping, or in various recipes!

Vegetable Chips:

Ingredients:

- Assorted vegetables (sweet potatoes, beets, zucchini, carrots, kale, etc.)
- Olive oil
- Salt and pepper to taste
- Optional: Seasonings like paprika, garlic powder, or dried herbs

Instructions:

1. Preheat the oven to 375°F (190°C).
2. Wash and peel (if necessary) the vegetables. Using a mandoline slicer or a sharp knife, slice the vegetables thinly and uniformly.
3. In a large bowl, toss the vegetable slices with olive oil to coat them evenly.
4. Season the slices with salt, pepper, and any optional seasonings of your choice.
5. Arrange the vegetable slices in a single layer on baking sheets lined with parchment paper. Ensure they are not overlapping to promote even cooking.
6. Bake in the preheated oven for 15-20 minutes or until the edges of the chips are golden brown and crisp. Keep an eye on them, as the cooking time may vary depending on the thickness of the slices.
7. Check the chips halfway through the cooking time and flip them for even crispiness.
8. Once the vegetable chips are done, remove them from the oven and let them cool on the baking sheets for a few minutes.
9. Transfer the chips to a wire rack to cool completely. They will continue to crisp up as they cool.
10. Enjoy your homemade Vegetable Chips as a wholesome snack or a crunchy accompaniment to your meals!

Cottage Cheese with Pineapple:

Ingredients:

- 1 cup cottage cheese
- 1 cup fresh pineapple chunks (or canned pineapple, drained)
- Honey or maple syrup for drizzling (optional)

Instructions:

1. Spoon the cottage cheese into a serving bowl.
2. Add fresh pineapple chunks on top of the cottage cheese.
3. If you desire a touch of sweetness, drizzle honey or maple syrup over the cottage cheese and pineapple.
4. Gently toss the ingredients together to combine.
5. Serve immediately and enjoy Cottage Cheese with Pineapple as a refreshing and protein-packed snack or light breakfast!
6. Optionally, you can sprinkle some nuts, seeds, or a dash of cinnamon for added flavor and texture.

Trail Mix:

Ingredients:

- 1 cup nuts (almonds, walnuts, cashews, etc.)
- 1 cup seeds (pumpkin seeds, sunflower seeds, etc.)
- 1 cup dried fruits (raisins, cranberries, apricots, etc.)
- 1 cup whole-grain cereal or pretzels
- 1/2 cup chocolate chips or dark chocolate chunks
- 1/2 cup coconut flakes (optional)
- 1/2 teaspoon salt (optional, for a sweet-savory mix)

Instructions:

1. In a large bowl, combine nuts, seeds, dried fruits, cereal, chocolate chips, and coconut flakes.
2. Optionally, sprinkle a bit of salt over the mix if you want a sweet-savory combination.
3. Toss all the ingredients together until evenly distributed.
4. Transfer the trail mix to an airtight container for storage.
5. Portion out the trail mix into snack-sized bags for convenient, grab-and-go servings.

6. Enjoy your Homemade Trail Mix as a nutritious and energy-boosting snack for hikes, workouts, or any time you need a quick bite!

Yogurt Parfait with Granola:

Ingredients:

- 1 cup Greek yogurt (plain or flavored)
- 1/2 cup granola (store-bought or homemade)
- 1/2 cup mixed berries (strawberries, blueberries, raspberries)
- 1 tablespoon honey or maple syrup
- Optional: Nuts or seeds (e.g., almonds, chia seeds)
- Optional: Fresh mint leaves for garnish

Instructions:

1. In a glass or a bowl, start by layering the bottom with a portion of Greek yogurt.
2. Add a layer of granola on top of the yogurt.
3. Spoon a layer of mixed berries over the granola.
4. Repeat the layers until you fill the glass or bowl, ending with a final layer of berries on top.
5. Drizzle honey or maple syrup over the parfait for sweetness.
6. Optionally, sprinkle nuts or seeds on the top for added crunch and nutrition.
7. Garnish with fresh mint leaves if desired.
8. Serve immediately and enjoy your delicious and nutritious Yogurt Parfait with Granola!
9. Customize your parfait with different fruits, flavored yogurt, or additional toppings to suit your preferences.

Edamame:

Ingredients:

- 2 cups edamame (fresh or frozen)
- 1 tablespoon soy sauce

- 1 teaspoon sesame oil
- 1 teaspoon sesame seeds (optional)
- Pinch of salt (optional)

Instructions:

1. If using frozen edamame, thaw them according to the package instructions.
2. Bring a pot of water to a boil.
3. Add edamame to the boiling water and cook for 4-5 minutes or until they are tender.
4. Drain the edamame and transfer them to a bowl.
5. In a small bowl, mix soy sauce and sesame oil.
6. Pour the soy sauce and sesame oil mixture over the edamame and toss until they are well-coated.
7. Optionally, sprinkle sesame seeds over the edamame for added flavor and texture.
8. Add a pinch of salt if desired, but be cautious as soy sauce already adds saltiness.
9. Serve the edamame warm as a tasty and protein-rich snack or appetizer.
10. Enjoy your Simple Edamame with a sprinkle of your favorite seasonings or as is!

Dark Chocolate and Almonds:

Ingredients:

- 1 cup dark chocolate chips or chopped dark chocolate
- 1 cup whole almonds

Instructions:

1. Line a baking sheet with parchment paper.
2. In a heatproof bowl, melt the dark chocolate using a double boiler or by microwaving in short 20-30 second bursts, stirring between each burst until smooth.
3. Once the chocolate is melted, remove it from the heat.
4. Add whole almonds to the melted dark chocolate, stirring until all the almonds are evenly coated.

5. Using a fork or a slotted spoon, lift each almond out of the chocolate, allowing excess chocolate to drip off, and place it on the prepared baking sheet.

6. Repeat the process until all almonds are coated and arranged on the baking sheet.

7. Allow the dark chocolate-covered almonds to cool and harden. You can speed up the process by placing them in the refrigerator for about 30 minutes.

8. Once hardened, break apart any almonds that may have stuck together.

9. Store the Dark Chocolate and Almonds in an airtight container at room temperature.

10. Enjoy this delightful combination of rich dark chocolate and crunchy almonds as a satisfying treat or a homemade gift!

Roasted Chickpeas:

Ingredients:

- 2 cans (15 oz each) chickpeas (garbanzo beans), drained and rinsed
- 2 tablespoons olive oil
- 1 teaspoon ground cumin
- 1 teaspoon smoked paprika
- 1/2 teaspoon garlic powder
- 1/2 teaspoon onion powder
- 1/4 teaspoon cayenne pepper (adjust to taste)
- Salt and black pepper to taste

Instructions:

1. Preheat the oven to 400°F (200°C).

2. Thoroughly rinse and drain the chickpeas. Pat them dry with a clean kitchen towel to remove excess moisture.

3. In a bowl, toss the chickpeas with olive oil until they are evenly coated.

4. In a small bowl, mix ground cumin, smoked paprika, garlic powder, onion powder, cayenne pepper, salt, and black pepper.

5. Sprinkle the spice mixture over the chickpeas and toss until they are well coated with the spices.

6. Spread the seasoned chickpeas in a single layer on a baking sheet lined with parchment paper.

7. Bake in the preheated oven for 25-30 minutes or until the chickpeas are crispy and golden brown. Shake the baking sheet or toss the chickpeas halfway through to ensure even roasting.

8. Remove from the oven and let the roasted chickpeas cool for a few minutes before serving.

9. Enjoy the Roasted Chickpeas as a crunchy and flavorful snack or as a topping for salads and soups!

Avocado Rice Cakes:

Ingredients:

- 2 rice cakes
- 1 ripe avocado
- Salt and pepper to taste
- Red pepper flakes (optional, for a bit of heat)
- Lemon juice (optional, for added freshness)
- Optional toppings: Cherry tomatoes, radish slices, microgreens, sesame seeds

Instructions:

1. Prepare Avocado Spread:
   - Cut the ripe avocado in half, remove the pit, and scoop the flesh into a bowl.
   - Mash the avocado with a fork until you achieve your desired consistency.
   - Season the mashed avocado with salt, pepper, and a squeeze of lemon juice if desired. Add red pepper flakes for a bit of heat.

2. Assemble the Avocado Rice Cakes:
   - Spread the mashed avocado evenly over the rice cakes.

3. Add Toppings:
   - Top the avocado-covered rice cakes with your choice of toppings. Sliced cherry tomatoes, radish slices, microgreens, or sesame seeds work well.
4. Season to Taste:
   - Sprinkle a bit more salt and pepper over the assembled avocado rice cakes if needed.
5. Serve:
   - Arrange the Avocado Rice Cakes on a plate and serve immediately.

Appetizer Ideas:

Caprese Skewers:

Ingredients:

- Fresh mozzarella balls (bocconcini)
- Cherry tomatoes
- Fresh basil leaves
- Balsamic glaze (store-bought or homemade)
- Extra virgin olive oil
- Salt and pepper to taste
- Optional: Wooden or metal skewers

Instructions:

1. Prepare Ingredients:
   - If using wooden skewers, soak them in water for at least 30 minutes to prevent burning.
2. Assemble Skewers:
   - Thread a fresh mozzarella ball, a cherry tomato, and a fresh basil leaf onto each skewer. Repeat until you fill the skewer.
3. Arrange:
   - Arrange the Caprese skewers on a serving platter or plate.

4. Season:
    - Drizzle extra virgin olive oil over the skewers.
    - Sprinkle with salt and pepper to taste.
5. Finish with Balsamic Glaze:
    - Drizzle balsamic glaze over the Caprese skewers for a sweet and tangy finish.

Stuffed Mushrooms:

Ingredients:

- 16-20 large button mushrooms, cleaned and stems removed
- 1/2 pound (225g) Italian sausage or ground chicken/turkey (optional)
- 1/2 cup breadcrumbs
- 1/2 cup grated Parmesan cheese
- 1/4 cup chopped fresh parsley
- 3 cloves garlic, minced
- 1/4 cup finely chopped onion
- Salt and black pepper to taste
- 2 tablespoons olive oil
- Optional: 1/4 cup shredded mozzarella cheese for topping

Instructions:

1. Prepare Mushrooms:
    - Preheat the oven to 375°F (190°C).
    - Clean the mushrooms and remove the stems. Place the mushroom caps on a baking sheet.
2. Prepare Filling:
    - If using sausage or ground meat, cook it in a skillet over medium heat until browned. Drain excess fat.

- o   In a bowl, combine the cooked meat (if using), breadcrumbs, Parmesan cheese, chopped parsley, minced garlic, chopped onion, salt, and pepper. Mix well.

3. Stuff Mushrooms:

- o   Using a small spoon, stuff each mushroom cap with the filling mixture, pressing it down slightly.

4. Drizzle with Olive Oil:

- o   Drizzle olive oil over the stuffed mushrooms. This adds moisture and helps with browning.

5. Bake:

- o   Bake in the preheated oven for 20-25 minutes or until the mushrooms are tender and the tops are golden brown.

6. Optional: Add Cheese:

- o   If desired, sprinkle shredded mozzarella cheese over each stuffed mushroom during the last 5 minutes of baking.

7. Serve:

- o   Remove from the oven and let them cool for a few minutes before serving.

Bruschetta:

Ingredients:

- 1 French baguette, sliced
- 4-5 ripe tomatoes, diced
- 3 cloves garlic, minced
- 1/4 cup fresh basil, chopped
- 2 tablespoons extra-virgin olive oil
- 1 teaspoon balsamic vinegar
- Salt and pepper to taste

Instructions:

1. Preheat your oven to 375°F (190°C).

2. Place the baguette slices on a baking sheet and toast in the oven for 5-7 minutes or until they are golden brown.

3. In a bowl, combine diced tomatoes, minced garlic, chopped basil, olive oil, and balsamic vinegar. Mix well.

4. Season the tomato mixture with salt and pepper to taste. Allow it to sit for a few minutes to let the flavors meld.

5. Once the baguette slices are toasted, remove them from the oven and let them cool slightly.

6. Spoon the tomato mixture generously onto each slice of toasted baguette.

7. Serve immediately and enjoy your delicious homemade bruschetta!

Spinach and Artichoke Dip:

Ingredients:

- 1 (10-ounce) package frozen chopped spinach, thawed and drained
- 1 (14-ounce) can artichoke hearts, drained and chopped
- 1/2 cup mayonnaise
- 1/2 cup sour cream
- 1 cup grated Parmesan cheese
- 1 cup shredded mozzarella cheese
- 1 teaspoon minced garlic
- 1/2 teaspoon onion powder
- 1/2 teaspoon dried oregano
- Salt and pepper to taste

Instructions:

1. Preheat your oven to 375°F (190°C).

2. In a large mixing bowl, combine the thawed and drained spinach with the chopped artichoke hearts.

3. Add mayonnaise, sour cream, Parmesan cheese, mozzarella cheese, minced garlic, onion powder, dried oregano, salt, and pepper to the bowl. Mix everything together until well combined.

4. Transfer the mixture to a baking dish, spreading it evenly.

5. Bake in the preheated oven for approximately 25-30 minutes or until the dip is hot and bubbly, and the top is lightly golden brown.

6. Remove from the oven and let it cool for a few minutes before serving.

7. Serve the spinach and artichoke dip with tortilla chips, sliced baguette, or vegetable sticks.

Cucumber Bites with Smoked Salmon:

Ingredients:

- 1 English cucumber, thinly sliced into rounds
- 4 ounces smoked salmon, sliced into bite-sized pieces
- 1/2 cup cream cheese, softened
- 2 tablespoons fresh dill, chopped
- 1 tablespoon capers, drained
- 1 tablespoon red onion, finely chopped
- Lemon zest (optional)
- Salt and black pepper to taste

Instructions:

1. In a bowl, mix the softened cream cheese with chopped dill, capers, and finely chopped red onion. Season with salt and black pepper to taste.

2. Lay out the cucumber slices on a serving platter or tray.

3. Spoon a small amount of the cream cheese mixture onto each cucumber slice.

4. Top each cucumber slice with a piece of smoked salmon.

5. Optional: Sprinkle a bit of lemon zest on top for a citrusy kick.

6. Garnish with additional dill for a fresh touch.

7. Arrange the cucumber bites on a serving platter and refrigerate until ready to serve.

8. Serve chilled and enjoy these elegant Cucumber Bites with Smoked Salmon as a delightful appetizer.

Guacamole with Veggie Dippers:

Guacamole Ingredients:

- 3 ripe avocados, peeled and pitted
- 1 small red onion, finely diced
- 1-2 tomatoes, diced
- 1-2 cloves garlic, minced
- 1 lime, juiced
- 1/4 cup fresh cilantro, chopped
- Salt and pepper to taste

Veggie Dippers:

- Carrot sticks
- Cucumber slices
- Bell pepper strips (assorted colors)
- Cherry tomatoes

Instructions:

1. In a bowl, mash the ripe avocados with a fork or potato masher until smooth, leaving some chunks for texture.

2. Add finely diced red onion, diced tomatoes, minced garlic, lime juice, and chopped cilantro to the mashed avocados. Mix well.

3. Season the guacamole with salt and pepper to taste. Adjust lime juice and salt as needed.

4. Prepare the veggie dippers by cutting carrots, cucumbers, bell peppers, and cherry tomatoes into sticks or slices.

5. Arrange the guacamole in a serving bowl and surround it with the assorted veggie dippers.

6. Serve immediately and enjoy this refreshing Guacamole with Veggie Dippers as a tasty and healthy snack or appetizer.

Deviled Eggs:

Ingredients:

- 6 large eggs
- 3 tablespoons mayonnaise
- 1 teaspoon Dijon mustard
- 1 teaspoon white vinegar
- Salt and pepper to taste
- Paprika for garnish
- Optional: Chopped fresh chives or parsley for garnish

Instructions:

1. Place the eggs in a single layer in a saucepan and cover them with water. Bring the water to a boil over medium-high heat.

2. Once boiling, reduce the heat to low, cover, and simmer for about 10-12 minutes.

3. Drain the hot water and transfer the eggs to a bowl of ice water to cool. Let them sit for a few minutes.

4. Once cooled, peel the eggs and cut them in half lengthwise. Carefully scoop out the yolks into a separate bowl.

5. Mash the egg yolks with a fork, and then add mayonnaise, Dijon mustard, white vinegar, salt, and pepper. Mix until smooth and well combined.

6. Spoon or pipe the yolk mixture back into the egg white halves.

7. Sprinkle paprika on top for a classic touch. Optionally, garnish with chopped fresh chives or parsley.

8. Refrigerate the deviled eggs for at least 30 minutes before serving to allow the flavors to meld.

9. Serve chilled and enjoy these classic Deviled Eggs as a delightful appetizer or party snack.

Mango Salsa with Tortilla Chips:

Ingredients:

- 2 ripe mangoes, peeled, pitted, and diced
- 1/2 red onion, finely chopped
- 1 red bell pepper, diced
- 1 jalapeño pepper, seeds removed and finely chopped
- 1/4 cup fresh cilantro, chopped
- Juice of 2 limes
- Salt and pepper to taste
- Tortilla chips for serving

Instructions:

1. In a bowl, combine the diced mangoes, finely chopped red onion, diced red bell pepper, chopped jalapeño pepper, and chopped cilantro.
2. Squeeze the juice of two limes over the mixture.
3. Season the salsa with salt and pepper to taste. Adjust lime juice and salt as needed.
4. Gently toss all the ingredients together until well combined.
5. Cover the bowl with plastic wrap and refrigerate for at least 30 minutes to let the flavors meld.
6. Just before serving, give the salsa a final gentle stir.
7. Serve the mango salsa in a bowl alongside tortilla chips.
8. Enjoy this refreshing Mango Salsa with Tortilla Chips as a flavorful appetizer or snack with a tropical twist.

Shrimp Cocktail:

Ingredients:

- 1 pound large shrimp, peeled and deveined

- 1 lemon, sliced
- Ice for serving

For the Cocktail Sauce:

- 1/2 cup ketchup
- 2 tablespoons horseradish (adjust to taste)
- 1 tablespoon fresh lemon juice
- 1 teaspoon Worcestershire sauce
- Hot sauce (optional, to taste)
- Salt and pepper to taste

Instructions:

1. Bring a large pot of water to a boil. Add a generous pinch of salt and the sliced lemon.
2. Once boiling, add the peeled and deveined shrimp to the pot. Cook for 2-3 minutes or until the shrimp turn pink and opaque.
3. Drain the shrimp immediately and transfer them to a bowl of ice water to cool rapidly. This helps retain their texture.
4. For the cocktail sauce, in a bowl, combine ketchup, horseradish, fresh lemon juice, Worcestershire sauce, and hot sauce if desired. Mix well.
5. Season the cocktail sauce with salt and pepper to taste. Adjust the horseradish and hot sauce according to your spice preference.
6. Once the shrimp are chilled, arrange them on a serving platter around a bowl of the cocktail sauce.
7. Serve the shrimp cocktail with additional lemon wedges and ice for a refreshing presentation.
8. Dip the shrimp in the cocktail sauce and enjoy this classic Shrimp Cocktail as an elegant appetizer.

Stuffed Bell Peppers:

Ingredients:

- 4 large bell peppers, halved and seeds removed
- 1 pound ground beef or turkey
- 1 cup cooked rice (white or brown)
- 1 cup black beans, drained and rinsed
- 1 cup corn kernels (fresh, frozen, or canned)
- 1 cup diced tomatoes
- 1 cup shredded cheese (cheddar, Monterey Jack, or a blend)
- 1/2 cup diced onion
- 2 cloves garlic, minced
- 1 teaspoon ground cumin
- 1 teaspoon chili powder
- Salt and pepper to taste
- Fresh cilantro or parsley for garnish (optional)

Instructions:

1. Preheat your oven to 375°F (190°C).
2. In a skillet over medium heat, cook the ground beef or turkey until browned. Drain excess fat if needed.
3. Add diced onion and minced garlic to the skillet and sauté until softened.
4. Stir in the cooked rice, black beans, corn, diced tomatoes, ground cumin, chili powder, salt, and pepper. Cook for a few minutes until the mixture is well combined and heated through.
5. Place the bell pepper halves in a baking dish.
6. Spoon the meat and rice mixture into each bell pepper half.
7. Top each stuffed pepper with shredded cheese.
8. Cover the baking dish with aluminum foil and bake in the preheated oven for 25-30 minutes or until the peppers are tender.
9. Remove the foil and bake for an additional 5-10 minutes until the cheese is melted and bubbly.
10. Garnish with fresh cilantro or parsley if desired.

Quinoa Salad Cups:

Ingredients:

For Quinoa Salad:

- 1 cup quinoa, rinsed and cooked according to package instructions
- 1 cup cherry tomatoes, halved
- 1 cucumber, diced
- 1 bell pepper (red, yellow, or orange), diced
- 1/2 red onion, finely chopped
- 1/4 cup fresh parsley, chopped
- Feta cheese crumbles (optional)
- Kalamata olives, sliced (optional)

For Dressing:

- 3 tablespoons extra-virgin olive oil
- 2 tablespoons red wine vinegar
- 1 teaspoon Dijon mustard
- 1 clove garlic, minced
- Salt and pepper to taste

For Salad Cups:

- Large lettuce leaves or mini cups (endive leaves or small tortilla cups)

Instructions:

1. Cook quinoa according to package instructions and let it cool to room temperature.
2. In a large bowl, combine the cooked quinoa, cherry tomatoes, cucumber, bell pepper, red onion, and chopped parsley.
3. If using, add Feta cheese crumbles and sliced Kalamata olives to the salad.
4. In a small bowl, whisk together the olive oil, red wine vinegar, Dijon mustard, minced garlic, salt, and pepper to create the dressing.
5. Pour the dressing over the quinoa salad and toss everything together until well coated.
6. Wash and prepare the lettuce leaves or mini cups for serving.

7. Spoon the quinoa salad into the lettuce leaves or mini cups, creating individual servings.

8. Optionally, garnish with additional parsley or a sprinkle of Feta cheese.

Mozzarella and Tomato Skewers:

Ingredients:

- Cherry tomatoes
- Fresh mozzarella balls (bocconcini)
- Fresh basil leaves
- Balsamic glaze (store-bought or homemade)
- Extra-virgin olive oil
- Salt and pepper to taste
- Wooden skewers

Instructions:

1. Rinse the cherry tomatoes and basil leaves.

2. Assemble your skewers by alternating cherry tomatoes, fresh mozzarella balls, and basil leaves.

3. Arrange the skewers on a serving platter or dish.

4. In a small bowl, mix together balsamic glaze and extra-virgin olive oil. You can adjust the ratio to suit your taste.

5. Drizzle the balsamic glaze and olive oil mixture over the mozzarella and tomato skewers.

6. Sprinkle with salt and pepper to taste.

7. Optionally, let the skewers marinate for a short time to enhance the flavors.

8. Serve the mozzarella and tomato skewers on the platter, allowing guests to drizzle extra balsamic glaze if desired.

Sweet Potato Rounds with Goat Cheese:

For Quinoa Salad:

- 1 cup quinoa, rinsed and cooked according to package instructions
- 1 cup cherry tomatoes, halved
- 1 cucumber, diced
- 1 bell pepper (red, yellow, or orange), diced
- 1/2 red onion, finely chopped
- 1/4 cup fresh parsley, chopped
- Feta cheese crumbles (optional)
- Kalamata olives, sliced (optional)

For Dressing:

- 3 tablespoons extra-virgin olive oil
- 2 tablespoons red wine vinegar
- 1 teaspoon Dijon mustard
- 1 clove garlic, minced
- Salt and pepper to taste

For Salad Cups:

- Large lettuce leaves or mini cups (endive leaves or small tortilla cups)

Instructions:

1. Cook quinoa according to package instructions and let it cool to room temperature.
2. In a large bowl, combine the cooked quinoa, cherry tomatoes, cucumber, bell pepper, red onion, and chopped parsley.
3. If using, add Feta cheese crumbles and sliced Kalamata olives to the salad.
4. In a small bowl, whisk together the olive oil, red wine vinegar, Dijon mustard, minced garlic, salt, and pepper to create the dressing.
5. Pour the dressing over the quinoa salad and toss everything together until well coated.
6. Wash and prepare the lettuce leaves or mini cups for serving.
7. Spoon the quinoa salad into the lettuce leaves or mini cups, creating individual servings.
8. Optionally, garnish with additional parsley or a sprinkle of Feta cheese.

Chicken Lettuce Wraps:

Ingredients:

For the Chicken Filling:

- 1 pound ground chicken
- 2 tablespoons soy sauce
- 1 tablespoon hoisin sauce
- 1 tablespoon sesame oil
- 1 tablespoon fresh ginger, minced
- 2 cloves garlic, minced
- 1 cup water chestnuts, finely chopped
- 1/4 cup green onions, sliced
- Salt and pepper to taste

For the Sauce:

- 2 tablespoons soy sauce
- 1 tablespoon hoisin sauce
- 1 tablespoon rice vinegar
- 1 teaspoon sesame oil

To Serve:

- Iceberg or butter lettuce leaves
- Additional sliced green onions for garnish
- Crushed peanuts (optional)

Instructions:

1. In a skillet or wok over medium-high heat, cook ground chicken until browned and cooked through.
2. In a small bowl, mix together soy sauce, hoisin sauce, and sesame oil. Add this mixture to the cooked chicken and stir.
3. Add minced ginger and garlic to the chicken mixture and sauté for 1-2 minutes until fragrant.

4. Stir in water chestnuts and sliced green onions. Cook for an additional 2-3 minutes.

5. Season with salt and pepper to taste.

6. In a separate bowl, whisk together the sauce ingredients: soy sauce, hoisin sauce, rice vinegar, and sesame oil.

7. Pour the sauce over the chicken mixture and stir until well combined. Cook for an additional 2-3 minutes.

8. Arrange lettuce leaves on a serving platter.

9. Spoon the chicken mixture into each lettuce leaf.

10. Garnish with additional sliced green onions and crushed peanuts if desired.

11. Serve immediately, allowing each person to wrap their own Chicken Lettuce Wraps.

Stuffed Avocado Halves:

Ingredients:

For the Filling:

- 2 ripe avocados, halved and pitted
- 1 cup cooked quinoa or rice
- 1 cup black beans, drained and rinsed
- 1 cup corn kernels (fresh, frozen, or canned)
- 1/2 cup cherry tomatoes, halved
- 1/4 cup red onion, finely chopped
- 1/4 cup fresh cilantro, chopped
- Juice of 1 lime
- Salt and pepper to taste

Optional Toppings:

- Greek yogurt or sour cream
- Salsa
- Shredded cheese

- Hot sauce

Instructions:

1. In a large bowl, combine cooked quinoa or rice, black beans, corn, cherry tomatoes, red onion, and chopped cilantro.
2. Squeeze lime juice over the mixture and toss until well combined.
3. Season with salt and pepper to taste. Adjust lime juice and salt as needed.
4. Scoop out a small portion of the avocado flesh to create a larger well for the filling.
5. Spoon the quinoa mixture into each avocado half, pressing down slightly.
6. Optional: Top with a dollop of Greek yogurt or sour cream, salsa, shredded cheese, and a drizzle of hot sauce.
7. Arrange the stuffed avocado halves on a serving platter.
8. Serve immediately, and enjoy these delicious and nutritious Stuffed Avocado Halves as a light meal or appetizer!

CHAPTER 7: SMOOTHIES AND BEVERAGES TO SUPPORT HEALING

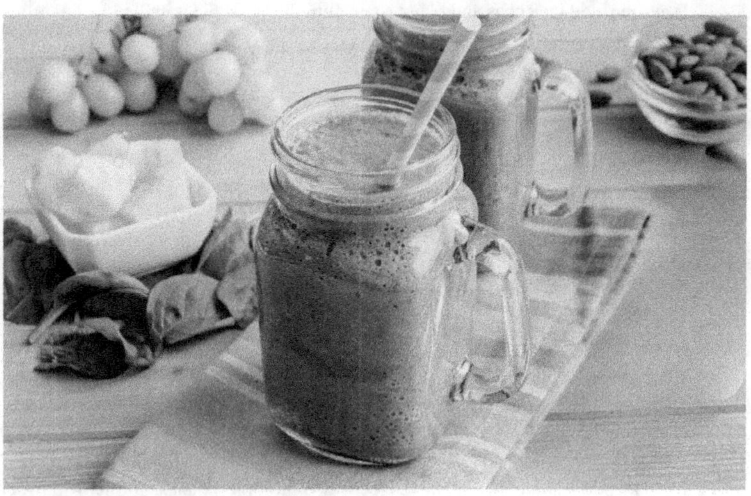

Green Detox Smoothie:

Ingredients:

- 1 cup fresh spinach leaves
- 1/2 cucumber, peeled and sliced
- 1 green apple, cored and chopped
- 1/2 lemon, juiced
- 1/2 inch ginger, peeled
- 1 cup coconut water or water
- Ice cubes (optional)

Instructions:

1. Place the fresh spinach leaves, cucumber slices, chopped green apple, peeled ginger, and lemon juice in a blender.

2. Add coconut water or water to the blender.

3. Blend on high speed until the ingredients are well combined and the smoothie reaches a creamy consistency.

4. If desired, add ice cubes and blend again until the smoothie is chilled.

5. Pour the green detox smoothie into a glass and enjoy immediately.

Anti-Inflammatory Berry Smoothie:

Ingredients:

- 1 cup mixed berries (blueberries, strawberries, raspberries)
- 1/2 cup pineapple chunks
- 1/2 teaspoon turmeric powder
- 1/2 teaspoon ginger, grated
- 1 tablespoon chia seeds
- 1 cup almond milk or any plant-based milk
- Ice cubes (optional)

Instructions:

1. In a blender, combine the mixed berries, pineapple chunks, turmeric powder, grated ginger, chia seeds, and almond milk.

2. Blend the ingredients on high speed until the smoothie is well mixed and reaches a creamy consistency.

3. If you prefer a colder smoothie, you can add ice cubes and blend again until they are incorporated.

4. Pour the anti-inflammatory berry smoothie into a glass.

5. Garnish with additional berries or a sprinkle of chia seeds if desired.

Immune-Boosting Citrus Smoothie:

Ingredients:

- 1 orange, peeled and segmented
- 1/2 grapefruit, peeled and segmented

- 1/2 lemon, juiced
- 1/2 inch ginger, peeled
- 1 banana
- 1 cup Greek yogurt or dairy-free yogurt for a plant-based option
- 1 tablespoon honey or maple syrup (optional)
- Ice cubes (optional)

Instructions:

1. Place the orange segments, grapefruit segments, lemon juice, peeled ginger, banana, Greek yogurt, and honey (if using) in a blender.
2. Blend on high speed until the ingredients are well combined and the smoothie reaches a creamy consistency.
3. If you like a colder smoothie, add ice cubes and blend again until they are incorporated.
4. Pour the immune-boosting citrus smoothie into a glass.
5. Garnish with a slice of citrus or a sprinkle of chia seeds if desired.

Digestive Health Smoothie:

Ingredients:

- 1 cup papaya, peeled, seeded, and chopped
- 1/2 cup pineapple chunks
- 1/2 banana
- 1/2 cup Greek yogurt or probiotic-rich yogurt
- 1 tablespoon chia seeds
- 1 tablespoon honey or maple syrup (optional)
- 1/2 teaspoon fresh mint leaves (optional)
- 1/2 cup coconut water or water
- Ice cubes (optional)

Instructions:

1. In a blender, combine the chopped papaya, pineapple chunks, banana, Greek yogurt, chia seeds, honey (if using), and fresh mint leaves.
2. Add coconut water or water to the blender.
3. Blend on high speed until the ingredients are well combined, and the smoothie reaches a creamy consistency.
4. If you prefer a colder smoothie, add ice cubes and blend again until they are incorporated.
5. Pour the digestive health smoothie into a glass.
6. Garnish with additional mint leaves or a sprinkle of chia seeds if desired.

Tropical Turmeric Smoothie:

Ingredients:

- 1 cup pineapple chunks
- 1/2 banana
- 1/2 cup mango chunks
- 1/2 teaspoon turmeric powder
- 1/2 teaspoon fresh ginger, grated
- 1 tablespoon chia seeds
- 1 cup coconut milk or almond milk
- 1 tablespoon honey or maple syrup (optional)
- Ice cubes (optional)

Instructions:

1. In a blender, combine the pineapple chunks, banana, mango chunks, turmeric powder, grated ginger, chia seeds, coconut milk, and honey (if using).
2. Blend on high speed until the ingredients are well combined, and the smoothie reaches a creamy consistency.
3. If you prefer a colder smoothie, add ice cubes and blend again until they are incorporated.
4. Pour the tropical turmeric smoothie into a glass.

5. Garnish with a slice of pineapple or a sprinkle of chia seeds if desired.

Protein-Packed Almond Butter Smoothie:

Ingredients:

- 1 banana
- 2 tablespoons almond butter
- 1/2 cup Greek yogurt or plant-based yogurt
- 1 cup almond milk
- 1 scoop vanilla protein powder
- 1 tablespoon chia seeds
- 1 tablespoon honey or maple syrup (optional)
- Ice cubes (optional)

Instructions:

1. In a blender, combine the banana, almond butter, Greek yogurt, almond milk, vanilla protein powder, chia seeds, and honey (if using).
2. Blend on high speed until the ingredients are well combined, and the smoothie reaches a creamy consistency.
3. If you prefer a colder smoothie, add ice cubes and blend again until they are incorporated.
4. Pour the protein-packed almond butter smoothie into a glass.
5. Garnish with a drizzle of almond butter or a sprinkle of chia seeds if desired.

Chia Seed and Berry Smoothie:

Ingredients:

- 1 cup mixed berries (strawberries, blueberries, raspberries)
- 1 banana
- 1 tablespoon chia seeds
- 1 cup almond milk or any plant-based milk
- 1 tablespoon honey or maple syrup (optional)

- Ice cubes (optional)

Instructions:

1. In a blender, combine the mixed berries, banana, chia seeds, almond milk, and honey (if using).
2. Blend on high speed until the ingredients are well combined, and the smoothie reaches a creamy consistency.
3. If you prefer a colder smoothie, add ice cubes and blend again until they are incorporated.
4. Pour the chia seed and berry smoothie into a glass.
5. Garnish with a few whole berries or a sprinkle of chia seeds if desired.

Hydrating Watermelon Mint Smoothie:

Ingredients:

- 2 cups watermelon, seeded and cubed
- 1/2 cucumber, peeled and sliced
- 1/4 cup fresh mint leaves
- 1 tablespoon lime juice
- 1 cup coconut water or water
- Ice cubes (optional)

Instructions:

1. In a blender, combine the watermelon cubes, sliced cucumber, fresh mint leaves, lime juice, and coconut water.
2. Blend on high speed until the ingredients are well combined, and the smoothie reaches a refreshing and hydrating consistency.
3. If you prefer a colder smoothie, add ice cubes and blend again until they are incorporated.
4. Pour the hydrating watermelon mint smoothie into a glass.
5. Garnish with a sprig of mint or a slice of cucumber if desired.

Recovery Banana and Peanut Butter Smoothie:

Ingredients:

- 2 ripe bananas
- 2 tablespoons peanut butter
- 1 cup Greek yogurt or plant-based yogurt
- 1 cup almond milk or any milk of your choice
- 1 tablespoon honey or maple syrup (optional)
- 1/2 teaspoon cinnamon
- 1/2 teaspoon vanilla extract
- Ice cubes (optional)

Instructions:

1. In a blender, combine the ripe bananas, peanut butter, Greek yogurt, almond milk, honey (if using), cinnamon, and vanilla extract.
2. Blend on high speed until the ingredients are well combined, and the smoothie reaches a creamy consistency.
3. If you prefer a colder smoothie, add ice cubes and blend again until they are incorporated.
4. Pour the recovery banana and peanut butter smoothie into a glass.
5. Garnish with a drizzle of peanut butter or a sprinkle of cinnamon if desired.

Pineapple Ginger Digestive Smoothie:

Ingredients:

- 1 cup pineapple chunks
- 1/2 banana
- 1/2 teaspoon fresh ginger, grated
- 1/2 cup Greek yogurt or plant-based yogurt
- 1 tablespoon chia seeds
- 1 tablespoon honey or maple syrup (optional)
- 1 cup coconut water or water

- Ice cubes (optional)

Instructions:

1. In a blender, combine the pineapple chunks, banana, grated ginger, Greek yogurt, chia seeds, honey (if using), and coconut water.

2. Blend on high speed until the ingredients are well combined, and the smoothie reaches a refreshing and digestive-friendly consistency.

3. If you prefer a colder smoothie, add ice cubes and blend again until they are incorporated.

4. Pour the pineapple ginger digestive smoothie into a glass.

5. Garnish with a slice of pineapple or a sprinkle of chia seeds if desired.

Cleansing Beet and Berry Smoothie:

Ingredients:

- 1/2 medium-sized beet, peeled and chopped
- 1/2 cup mixed berries (blueberries, raspberries, strawberries)
- 1/2 cucumber, peeled and sliced
- 1/2 lemon, juiced
- 1 tablespoon chia seeds
- 1 cup coconut water or water
- 1 tablespoon honey or maple syrup (optional)
- Ice cubes (optional)

Instructions:

1. In a blender, combine the chopped beet, mixed berries, sliced cucumber, lemon juice, chia seeds, honey (if using), and coconut water.

2. Blend on high speed until the ingredients are well combined, and the smoothie reaches a vibrant and cleansing consistency.

3. If you prefer a colder smoothie, add ice cubes and blend again until they are incorporated.

4. Pour the cleansing beet and berry smoothie into a glass.

5. Garnish with a few berries or a sprinkle of chia seeds if desired.

Probiotic Mango Lassi Smoothie:

Ingredients:

- 1 cup ripe mango, peeled and chopped
- 1 cup plain yogurt or Greek yogurt
- 1/2 cup milk or a dairy-free alternative
- 1 tablespoon honey or maple syrup
- 1/2 teaspoon ground cardamom
- 1/2 teaspoon vanilla extract
- A pinch of salt
- Ice cubes (optional)

Instructions:

1. In a blender, combine the chopped mango, yogurt, milk, honey, ground cardamom, vanilla extract, and a pinch of salt.
2. Blend on high speed until the ingredients are well combined, and the smoothie reaches a creamy consistency.
3. If you prefer a colder smoothie, add ice cubes and blend again until they are incorporated.
4. Pour the probiotic mango lassi smoothie into a glass.
5. Optionally, garnish with a sprinkle of ground cardamom or a few mango cubes.

Chocolate Avocado Bliss Smoothie:

Ingredients:

- 1 ripe avocado, peeled and pitted
- 1 banana
- 2 tablespoons cocoa powder
- 1 tablespoon almond butter
- 1 cup almond milk or any milk of your choice

- 1-2 tablespoons honey or maple syrup (adjust to taste)
- 1/2 teaspoon vanilla extract
- Ice cubes (optional)

Instructions:

1. In a blender, combine the ripe avocado, banana, cocoa powder, almond butter, almond milk, honey, and vanilla extract.
2. Blend on high speed until the ingredients are well combined, and the smoothie reaches a creamy and chocolatey consistency.
3. If you prefer a colder smoothie, add ice cubes and blend again until they are incorporated.
4. Taste the smoothie and adjust sweetness if needed by adding more honey or maple syrup.
5. Pour the chocolate avocado bliss smoothie into a glass.
6. Optionally, garnish with a sprinkle of cocoa powder or a few slices of banana.

Anti-Stress Lavender Blueberry Smoothie:

Ingredients:

- 1 cup blueberries (fresh or frozen)
- 1/2 banana
- 1/2 cup Greek yogurt or plant-based yogurt
- 1/2 teaspoon dried lavender buds (culinary-grade)
- 1 tablespoon honey or maple syrup
- 1/2 teaspoon vanilla extract
- 1 cup almond milk or any milk of your choice
- Ice cubes (optional)

Instructions:

1. In a blender, combine the blueberries, banana, Greek yogurt, dried lavender buds, honey, vanilla extract, and almond milk.

2. Blend on high speed until the ingredients are well combined, and the smoothie reaches a smooth and calming consistency.

3. If you prefer a colder smoothie, add ice cubes and blend again until they are incorporated.

4. Pour the anti-stress lavender blueberry smoothie into a glass.

5. Optionally, garnish with a few extra blueberries or a sprinkle of dried lavender buds.

Post-Surgery Protein Smoothie:

Ingredients:

- 1 cup unsweetened almond milk or any milk of your choice
- 1/2 cup Greek yogurt or plant-based yogurt
- 1/2 banana
- 1/2 cup mango chunks
- 1 scoop vanilla protein powder
- 1 tablespoon almond butter
- 1 tablespoon chia seeds
- 1 tablespoon honey or maple syrup (optional)
- Ice cubes (optional)

Instructions:

1. In a blender, combine the almond milk, Greek yogurt, banana, mango chunks, vanilla protein powder, almond butter, chia seeds, and honey (if using).

2. Blend on high speed until the ingredients are well combined, and the smoothie reaches a creamy and protein-rich consistency.

3. If you prefer a colder smoothie, add ice cubes and blend again until they are incorporated.

4. Pour the post-surgery protein smoothie into a glass.

5. Optionally, garnish with a drizzle of almond butter or a sprinkle of chia seeds.

Turmeric Golden Milk:

Ingredients:

- 1 cup milk (dairy or plant-based)
- 1/2 teaspoon ground turmeric
- 1/4 teaspoon ground cinnamon
- 1/4 teaspoon ground ginger
- 1 tablespoon honey or maple syrup (adjust to taste)
- 1/2 teaspoon coconut oil (optional for added richness)
- A pinch of black pepper (enhances turmeric absorption)

Instructions:

1. In a small saucepan, heat the milk over medium heat until it's warm but not boiling.
2. Add the ground turmeric, ground cinnamon, ground ginger, honey (or maple syrup), coconut oil (if using), and a pinch of black pepper to the warm milk.
3. Whisk the ingredients continuously while heating until the mixture is well combined and heated through. Do not let it boil.
4. Once the turmeric golden milk is well mixed and warm, remove it from the heat.
5. Pour the golden milk into a mug and enjoy immediately.

Ginger Lemonade:

Ingredients:

- 4 cups water
- 1/2 cup freshly squeezed lemon juice (about 3-4 lemons)
- 1/4 cup honey or maple syrup (adjust to taste)
- 1 tablespoon fresh ginger, grated
- Ice cubes
- Lemon slices and fresh mint for garnish (optional)

Instructions:

1. In a small saucepan, combine 1 cup of water with the grated ginger. Bring it to a simmer over medium heat, then let it simmer for about 5 minutes. Remove from heat and let it cool slightly.

2. In a pitcher, combine the remaining 3 cups of water, freshly squeezed lemon juice, honey (or maple syrup), and the ginger-infused water.

3. Stir well to ensure the sweetener is dissolved.

4. Refrigerate the ginger lemonade for at least 1-2 hours to allow the flavors to meld.

5. Before serving, strain the ginger pieces if desired.

6. Pour the ginger lemonade over ice cubes in glasses.

7. Garnish with lemon slices and fresh mint if you like.

Green Tea with Mint:

Ingredients:

- 2 green tea bags or 2 teaspoons loose green tea leaves
- 2 cups water
- Fresh mint leaves
- Honey or sweetener of choice (optional)
- Ice cubes (optional)

Instructions:

1. Boil 2 cups of water.

2. Place the green tea bags or loose green tea leaves in a teapot or heatproof container.

3. Pour the hot water over the tea bags or leaves.

4. Allow the tea to steep for about 3-5 minutes, or until you achieve your desired strength. Be cautious not to over-steep, as green tea can become bitter.

5. While the tea is still hot, add fresh mint leaves to the pot or container. You can bruise the mint leaves slightly to release more flavor.

6. Optionally, add honey or your preferred sweetener to the hot tea, stirring until dissolved.

7. Strain the tea to remove the tea bags or leaves and mint leaves.

8. If you prefer iced tea, let the tea cool to room temperature and then refrigerate. You can serve it over ice cubes.

9. Garnish with fresh mint leaves when serving.

Chamomile Lavender Tea:

Ingredients:

- 2 chamomile tea bags or 2 teaspoons dried chamomile flowers
- 1 teaspoon dried lavender buds (culinary-grade)
- 2 cups hot water
- Honey or sweetener of choice (optional)
- Lemon slices for garnish (optional)

Instructions:

1. Boil 2 cups of water.

2. Place the chamomile tea bags or chamomile flowers and dried lavender buds in a teapot or heatproof container.

3. Pour the hot water over the tea bags or flowers and lavender.

4. Allow the tea to steep for about 5-7 minutes, or until you achieve your desired strength.

5. While the tea is still hot, you can add honey or your preferred sweetener, stirring until dissolved.

6. Strain the tea to remove the tea bags or flowers and lavender buds.

7. Pour the chamomile lavender tea into cups.

8. Optionally, garnish with a slice of lemon.

Bone Broth:

Ingredients:

- 2-3 pounds of beef or chicken bones (with marrow and knuckles for added collagen)
- 2 carrots, roughly chopped
- 2 celery stalks, roughly chopped
- 1 onion, quartered
- 4 cloves garlic, smashed
- 2 tablespoons apple cider vinegar
- Fresh herbs (such as parsley, thyme, or bay leaves)
- Salt and pepper to taste
- Water (enough to cover the bones)

Instructions:

1. Preheat your oven to 400°F (200°C).
2. Place the bones on a baking sheet and roast them in the oven for about 30 minutes. This helps enhance the flavor of the broth.
3. Transfer the roasted bones to a large stockpot.
4. Add chopped carrots, celery, onion, and smashed garlic to the pot.
5. Pour in enough water to cover the bones (about 4 quarts or liters).
6. Add apple cider vinegar, fresh herbs, salt, and pepper.
7. Bring the mixture to a boil, then reduce the heat to low. Skim off any foam that rises to the surface.
8. Cover the pot and let it simmer on low heat for at least 4-6 hours (or up to 24 hours for a richer broth). The longer you simmer, the more nutrients and collagen will be extracted from the bones.
9. Strain the broth through a fine-mesh sieve or cheesecloth into a large bowl or another pot to remove solids.
10. Let the broth cool, then refrigerate. Once cooled, the fat will rise to the top and solidify, making it easier to remove if desired.
11. Use the bone broth as a base for soups, stews, or enjoy it on its own.

Cucumber Basil Infused Water:

Ingredients:

- 1 cucumber, thinly sliced
- Handful of fresh basil leaves
- 1-2 liters of water (filtered or still)
- Ice cubes (optional)

Instructions:

1. Wash the cucumber thoroughly and slice it thinly.
2. Rinse the fresh basil leaves.
3. In a large pitcher, combine the cucumber slices and basil leaves.
4. Fill the pitcher with 1-2 liters of water, depending on your desired concentration.
5. Add ice cubes if you prefer a chilled infusion.
6. Stir the ingredients gently with a long spoon.
7. Let the cucumber and basil infuse into the water for at least 1-2 hours. For a stronger flavor, you can refrigerate the pitcher overnight.
8. Pour the infused water into glasses, and if desired, garnish with additional cucumber slices or basil leaves.

Hibiscus Iced Tea:

Ingredients:

- 2 hibiscus tea bags or 2 tablespoons dried hibiscus flowers
- 4 cups water
- 1-2 tablespoons honey or sweetener of choice (adjust to taste)
- Ice cubes
- Orange slices or mint leaves for garnish (optional)

Instructions:

1. Boil 4 cups of water.
2. Place the hibiscus tea bags or hibiscus flowers in a heatproof container.
3. Pour the boiling water over the tea bags or flowers.

4. Allow the hibiscus tea to steep for about 5-7 minutes, or until you achieve your desired strength.

5. Remove the tea bags or strain out the hibiscus flowers.

6. Add honey or your preferred sweetener to the hot tea, stirring until dissolved.

7. Let the hibiscus tea cool to room temperature.

8. Refrigerate the tea for at least 1-2 hours to chill.

9. Fill glasses with ice cubes and pour the chilled hibiscus tea over the ice.

10. Optionally, garnish with orange slices or mint leaves.

Peppermint Tea:

Ingredients:

- 1-2 peppermint tea bags or 1 tablespoon dried peppermint leaves
- 1 cup boiling water
- Honey or sweetener of choice (optional)
- Fresh mint leaves for garnish (optional)

Instructions:

1. Place the peppermint tea bag or dried peppermint leaves in a teapot or heatproof container.

2. Pour 1 cup of boiling water over the tea bag or leaves.

3. Allow the peppermint tea to steep for about 5-7 minutes, or until you achieve your desired strength.

4. Remove the tea bag or strain out the peppermint leaves.

5. Add honey or your preferred sweetener to the hot tea, stirring until dissolved (if desired).

6. Pour the peppermint tea into a cup.

7. Optionally, garnish with fresh mint leaves.

Pomegranate Elixir:

Ingredients:

- 1 cup pomegranate juice (freshly squeezed or store-bought)
- 1 tablespoon honey or maple syrup (adjust to taste)
- 1-2 teaspoons fresh lemon juice
- 1-2 tablespoons chia seeds (optional, for added texture)
- Ice cubes
- Pomegranate arils for garnish (optional)
- Mint leaves for garnish (optional)

Instructions:

1. In a glass or pitcher, combine the pomegranate juice, honey or maple syrup, and fresh lemon juice.
2. Stir well until the sweetener is fully dissolved.
3. Optionally, add chia seeds to the mixture, stirring to combine. Let it sit for a few minutes to allow the chia seeds to absorb liquid and create a gel-like texture.
4. Fill glasses with ice cubes.
5. Pour the pomegranate elixir over the ice.
6. Optionally, garnish with pomegranate arils and mint leaves for a decorative touch.
7. Stir before drinking to distribute the flavors evenly.

Aloe Vera Coconut Water Refresher:

Ingredients:

- 1 cup coconut water
- 2 tablespoons fresh aloe vera gel (extracted from the leaf)
- 1 tablespoon honey or agave syrup (optional)
- 1/2 teaspoon lime juice
- Ice cubes
- Mint leaves for garnish (optional)

Instructions:

1. Cut an aloe vera leaf, wash it thoroughly, and extract 2 tablespoons of fresh aloe vera gel.
2. In a glass, combine the coconut water, fresh aloe vera gel, honey or agave syrup (if using), and lime juice.
3. Stir well to ensure the ingredients are thoroughly mixed.
4. Add ice cubes to the glass.
5. Optionally, garnish with fresh mint leaves for added freshness.
6. Stir again before serving to incorporate the flavors.

Carrot Ginger Wellness Juice:

Ingredients:

- 4 medium carrots, washed and chopped
- 1-inch piece of fresh ginger, peeled
- 1 apple, cored and chopped
- 1/2 lemon, peeled
- 1-2 tablespoons honey or maple syrup (optional)
- 2 cups water
- Ice cubes (optional)

Instructions:

1. In a blender, combine the chopped carrots, fresh ginger, chopped apple, and peeled lemon.
2. Add water to the blender.
3. Blend on high speed until the ingredients are well combined and the juice reaches a smooth consistency.
4. Strain the juice using a fine-mesh sieve or cheesecloth to remove the pulp.
5. If desired, add honey or maple syrup to the strained juice and stir until dissolved.
6. Pour the carrot ginger wellness juice into glasses.
7. Optionally, add ice cubes for a chilled refreshment.

Matcha Latte:

Ingredients:

- 1 teaspoon matcha powder
- 1-2 teaspoons honey or sweetener of choice (adjust to taste)
- 1 cup milk (dairy or plant-based)
- Hot water (not boiling)
- Optional: Vanilla extract or flavored syrup for extra sweetness
- Optional: Whisk or frother for better matcha blending
- Optional: Matcha whisk or spoon for traditional preparation

Instructions:

1. In a cup, add the matcha powder.
2. Pour a small amount of hot water into the cup with the matcha powder. Whisk or stir well to create a smooth matcha paste.
3. Heat the milk in a saucepan or microwave until warm but not boiling.
4. Pour the warm milk over the matcha paste in the cup.
5. Add honey or sweetener to the matcha latte and stir until well combined.
6. Optional: Add a few drops of vanilla extract or flavored syrup for extra sweetness.
7. Use a whisk or frother to froth the matcha latte until a layer of foam forms on top.
8. Alternatively, you can whisk the matcha traditionally using a matcha whisk or spoon by vigorously stirring in a "W" or "M" motion until frothy.
9. Enjoy your matcha latte immediately.

Lemon Turmeric Infused Water:

Ingredients:

- 1 lemon, thinly sliced
- 1 teaspoon fresh turmeric, peeled and sliced (or 1/2 teaspoon ground turmeric)
- 2-3 cups water
- Ice cubes
- Optional: Honey or agave syrup for sweetness

- Optional: Fresh mint leaves for garnish

Instructions:

1. Wash the lemon thoroughly and slice it thinly.
2. Peel and slice the fresh turmeric. If using ground turmeric, skip this step.
3. In a pitcher, combine the lemon slices and turmeric.
4. Pour 2-3 cups of water over the lemon and turmeric.
5. Add ice cubes to the pitcher for a chilled infusion.
6. Optionally, add honey or agave syrup to sweeten the infused water. Stir until the sweetener is dissolved.
7. Let the lemon turmeric infused water sit for at least 15-20 minutes to allow the flavors to meld.
8. Pour the infused water into glasses.
9. Optionally, garnish with fresh mint leaves for added freshness.

Berry Hibiscus Kombucha:

Ingredients:

- 1 cup mixed berries (strawberries, blueberries, raspberries)
- 2 hibiscus tea bags or 2 tablespoons dried hibiscus flowers
- 1/4 cup honey or agave syrup
- 1 gallon brewed and cooled black or green tea
- 1 SCOBY (Symbiotic Culture Of Bacteria and Yeast)
- 1-2 cups starter kombucha (from a previous batch or store-bought)
- Glass fermentation jar

Instructions:

1. Brew a gallon of black or green tea and let it cool to room temperature.
2. In a small saucepan, combine the mixed berries and hibiscus tea bags or hibiscus flowers. Add 1/4 cup honey or agave syrup.
3. Simmer the berry and hibiscus mixture over low heat for about 10 minutes, mashing the berries to release their juices. Allow the mixture to cool.

4. Strain the berry and hibiscus mixture to remove solids, leaving a concentrated liquid.

5. In a large fermentation jar, combine the cooled tea, strained berry-hibiscus concentrate, SCOBY, and starter kombucha.

6. Cover the jar with a clean cloth and secure it with a rubber band. This allows the kombucha to breathe while keeping contaminants out.

7. Place the jar in a dark, warm place for 7-14 days, depending on your desired level of fermentation. Taste it periodically until it reaches the desired flavor.

8. Once the kombucha is ready, remove the SCOBY and reserve 1-2 cups of the liquid as a starter for your next batch.

9. Bottle the remaining kombucha, adding a few berries to each bottle if desired.

10. Seal the bottles tightly and let them sit at room temperature for 2-3 more days for carbonation.

11. Refrigerate the bottles to halt the fermentation process.

12. Serve the berry hibiscus kombucha chilled and enjoy!

Minty Pineapple Cooler:

Ingredients:

- 2 cups fresh pineapple chunks
- 1/4 cup fresh mint leaves
- 1 tablespoon honey or agave syrup
- 2 cups cold water
- Ice cubes
- Mint sprigs for garnish (optional)
- Pineapple slices for garnish (optional)

Instructions:

1. In a blender, combine fresh pineapple chunks, mint leaves, honey or agave syrup, and cold water.

2. Blend on high speed until the ingredients are well combined, and the mixture reaches a smooth consistency.

3. Strain the mixture through a fine-mesh sieve or cheesecloth to remove pulp and mint leaves.

4. Pour the strained pineapple-mint mixture into a pitcher.

5. Add ice cubes to the pitcher for a refreshing chill.

6. Stir well to mix in the ice.

7. Pour the minty pineapple cooler into glasses.

8. Optionally, garnish with mint sprigs or pineapple slices for an extra touch.

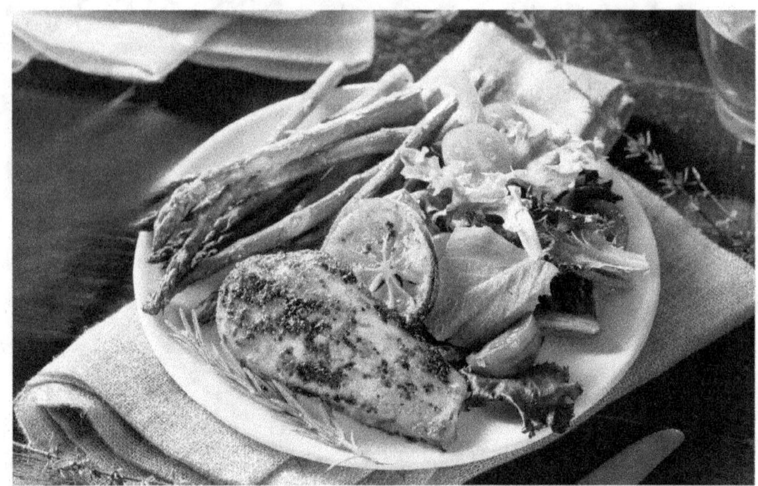

Classic Caesar Salad:

Ingredients:

For the Caesar Dressing:

- 1/2 cup mayonnaise
- 2 tablespoons grated Parmesan cheese
- 1 tablespoon Dijon mustard
- 2 cloves garlic, minced
- 1 tablespoon anchovy paste (optional)
- 1 tablespoon fresh lemon juice
- 1 teaspoon Worcestershire sauce
- Salt and black pepper to taste

For the Salad:

- 1 large head of romaine lettuce, washed and torn into bite-sized pieces

* 1 cup croutons
* 1/2 cup grated Parmesan cheese
* Lemon wedges for garnish (optional)

Instructions:

1. In a bowl, whisk together mayonnaise, grated Parmesan, Dijon mustard, minced garlic, anchovy paste (if using), fresh lemon juice, and Worcestershire sauce.
2. Season the dressing with salt and black pepper to taste. Adjust the ingredients as needed for your preferred flavor.
3. In a large salad bowl, combine the torn romaine lettuce with croutons.
4. Pour the Caesar dressing over the lettuce and croutons. Toss the salad to ensure even coating.
5. Sprinkle grated Parmesan cheese over the salad and toss again.
6. Serve the classic Caesar salad on individual plates or in a large serving bowl.
7. Optionally, garnish with additional croutons and lemon wedges.

Caprese Salad:

Ingredients:

* 4 large ripe tomatoes, sliced
* 200g fresh mozzarella cheese, sliced
* Fresh basil leaves
* Extra virgin olive oil
* Balsamic glaze or balsamic reduction
* Salt and black pepper to taste

Instructions:

1. Arrange the tomato and mozzarella slices alternately on a serving platter.
2. Tuck fresh basil leaves between the tomato and mozzarella slices.
3. Drizzle extra virgin olive oil over the salad.
4. Sprinkle salt and black pepper to taste.

5. Optionally, drizzle balsamic glaze or balsamic reduction over the salad for added flavor.

6. Serve the Caprese salad immediately, allowing the flavors to meld.

Quinoa and Vegetable Salad:

Ingredients:

For the Salad:

- 1 cup quinoa, rinsed
- 2 cups water or vegetable broth
- 1 cup cherry tomatoes, halved
- 1 cucumber, diced
- 1 bell pepper (any color), diced
- 1/2 red onion, finely chopped
- 1/4 cup Kalamata olives, sliced
- 1/4 cup feta cheese, crumbled (optional)
- Fresh parsley, chopped for garnish

For the Dressing:

- 1/4 cup extra virgin olive oil
- 2 tablespoons red wine vinegar
- 1 teaspoon Dijon mustard
- 1 clove garlic, minced
- Salt and black pepper to taste

Instructions:

1. In a saucepan, combine quinoa and water or vegetable broth. Bring to a boil, then reduce heat to low, cover, and simmer for 15-20 minutes, or until the quinoa is cooked and water is absorbed. Fluff with a fork and let it cool.

2. In a large salad bowl, combine the cooked quinoa, cherry tomatoes, cucumber, bell pepper, red onion, olives, and feta cheese.

3. In a small bowl or jar, whisk together the olive oil, red wine vinegar, Dijon mustard, minced garlic, salt, and black pepper to create the dressing.

4. Pour the dressing over the quinoa and vegetable mixture. Toss to coat the salad evenly.

5. Garnish the quinoa and vegetable salad with chopped fresh parsley.

6. Refrigerate for at least 30 minutes before serving to allow the flavors to meld.

Greek Salad:

Ingredients:

For the Salad:

- 4 cups cherry tomatoes, halved
- 1 cucumber, diced
- 1 red bell pepper, diced
- 1 green bell pepper, diced
- 1/2 red onion, thinly sliced
- 1 cup Kalamata olives, pitted
- 1 cup feta cheese, crumbled
- Fresh oregano leaves for garnish (optional)

For the Dressing:

- 1/4 cup extra virgin olive oil
- 2 tablespoons red wine vinegar
- 1 teaspoon dried oregano
- 1 clove garlic, minced
- Salt and black pepper to taste

Instructions:

1. In a large salad bowl, combine cherry tomatoes, cucumber, red bell pepper, green bell pepper, red onion, olives, and crumbled feta cheese.

2. In a small bowl or jar, whisk together olive oil, red wine vinegar, dried oregano, minced garlic, salt, and black pepper to create the dressing.

3. Pour the dressing over the salad ingredients.

4. Toss the Greek salad gently to ensure the vegetables are coated with the dressing.

5. Garnish with fresh oregano leaves if desired.

6. Refrigerate the salad for at least 30 minutes before serving to enhance the flavors.

7. Serve chilled and enjoy this classic Greek salad!

Mango Avocado Salad:

Ingredients:

For the Salad:

- 2 ripe mangoes, peeled, pitted, and diced
- 2 avocados, peeled, pitted, and diced
- 1 cup cherry tomatoes, halved
- 1/4 cup red onion, finely chopped
- 1/4 cup fresh cilantro, chopped
- 1 jalapeño, seeded and finely chopped (optional)
- Mixed salad greens (e.g., arugula or spinach)

For the Dressing:

- 2 tablespoons lime juice
- 2 tablespoons extra virgin olive oil
- 1 teaspoon honey or agave syrup
- Salt and black pepper to taste

Instructions:

1. In a large salad bowl, combine diced mangoes, diced avocados, cherry tomatoes, red onion, cilantro, and jalapeño (if using).

2. In a small bowl, whisk together lime juice, olive oil, honey or agave syrup, salt, and black pepper to create the dressing.

3. Pour the dressing over the mango and avocado salad.

4. Gently toss the salad to ensure even coating.

5. Arrange mixed salad greens on a serving platter or individual plates.

6. Spoon the mango avocado mixture over the bed of salad greens.

7. Serve immediately and enjoy this refreshing and tropical mango avocado salad!

Kale and Cranberry Salad:

Ingredients:

For the Salad:

- 6 cups kale, stems removed and leaves chopped
- 1 cup dried cranberries
- 1/2 cup feta cheese, crumbled
- 1/2 cup walnuts, chopped
- 1 apple, thinly sliced

For the Dressing:

- 1/4 cup extra virgin olive oil
- 2 tablespoons apple cider vinegar
- 1 tablespoon Dijon mustard
- 1 tablespoon honey or maple syrup
- Salt and black pepper to taste

Instructions:

1. In a large bowl, combine chopped kale, dried cranberries, crumbled feta cheese, chopped walnuts, and thinly sliced apple.

2. In a small bowl or jar, whisk together olive oil, apple cider vinegar, Dijon mustard, honey or maple syrup, salt, and black pepper to create the dressing.

3. Pour the dressing over the kale and cranberry salad.

4. Toss the salad gently to ensure the ingredients are evenly coated with the dressing.

5. Let the salad sit for a few minutes to allow the kale to soften slightly.

6. Serve the kale and cranberry salad as a side dish or a light meal.

Spinach and Strawberry Salad:

Ingredients:

For the Salad:

- 6 cups fresh baby spinach, washed and dried
- 2 cups strawberries, hulled and sliced
- 1/2 cup red onion, thinly sliced
- 1/2 cup feta cheese, crumbled
- 1/2 cup candied pecans or walnuts, chopped (optional)

For the Dressing:

- 1/4 cup balsamic vinegar
- 2 tablespoons extra virgin olive oil
- 1 tablespoon honey or maple syrup
- 1 teaspoon Dijon mustard
- Salt and black pepper to taste

Instructions:

1. In a large salad bowl, combine fresh baby spinach, sliced strawberries, thinly sliced red onion, crumbled feta cheese, and candied pecans or walnuts (if using).
2. In a small bowl or jar, whisk together balsamic vinegar, olive oil, honey or maple syrup, Dijon mustard, salt, and black pepper to create the dressing.
3. Pour the dressing over the spinach and strawberry salad.
4. Toss the salad gently to ensure the ingredients are evenly coated with the dressing.
5. Serve the spinach and strawberry salad immediately as a refreshing side or light meal.

Roasted Vegetable Salad:

Ingredients:

For the Roasted Vegetables:

- 2 cups cherry tomatoes, halved
- 1 zucchini, sliced
- 1 bell pepper (any color), sliced
- 1 red onion, sliced

- 2 tablespoons olive oil
- 2 teaspoons dried thyme
- Salt and black pepper to taste

For the Salad:

- Mixed salad greens (e.g., arugula or spinach)
- 1/2 cup crumbled feta cheese
- Balsamic vinaigrette dressing

Optional Additions:

- Roasted sweet potatoes or butternut squash
- Avocado slices
- Toasted pine nuts or walnuts

Instructions:

1. Preheat the oven to 400°F (200°C).
2. In a large mixing bowl, toss cherry tomatoes, sliced zucchini, bell pepper, and red onion with olive oil, dried thyme, salt, and black pepper until well coated.
3. Spread the vegetables on a baking sheet lined with parchment paper.
4. Roast in the preheated oven for 20-25 minutes or until the vegetables are tender and slightly caramelized. Stir once or twice during roasting.
5. Remove the roasted vegetables from the oven and let them cool slightly.
6. In a salad bowl, combine mixed salad greens with the roasted vegetables.
7. Sprinkle crumbled feta cheese over the salad.
8. Drizzle balsamic vinaigrette dressing over the salad and toss gently to combine.
9. If desired, add optional additions like roasted sweet potatoes or butternut squash, avocado slices, or toasted nuts.
10. Serve the roasted vegetable salad as a hearty and flavorful side or a light meal.

Cobb Salad:

Ingredients:

For the Salad:

- 6 cups mixed salad greens (e.g., Romaine lettuce, spinach)
- 2 cups cooked and diced chicken breast
- 1 cup cherry tomatoes, halved
- 1 cup cucumber, diced
- 1 cup avocado, diced
- 1/2 cup red onion, finely chopped
- 1/2 cup blue cheese, crumbled
- 4 hard-boiled eggs, sliced

For the Dressing:

- 1/4 cup red wine vinegar
- 1/2 cup extra virgin olive oil
- 1 teaspoon Dijon mustard
- 1 clove garlic, minced
- 1 teaspoon honey or maple syrup
- Salt and black pepper to taste

Instructions:

1. In a large salad bowl, arrange mixed salad greens as the base.
2. Create rows of diced chicken, cherry tomatoes, cucumber, diced avocado, chopped red onion, crumbled blue cheese, and sliced hard-boiled eggs on top of the greens.
3. In a small bowl or jar, whisk together red wine vinegar, olive oil, Dijon mustard, minced garlic, honey or maple syrup, salt, and black pepper to create the dressing.
4. Drizzle the dressing over the Cobb salad.
5. Serve the Cobb salad immediately, allowing each person to mix the ingredients and dressing according to their preference.

Asian Sesame Chicken Salad:

Ingredients:

For the Salad:

- 2 cups shredded cooked chicken breast

- 6 cups mixed salad greens (e.g., Napa cabbage, romaine lettuce, shredded carrots)
- 1 cup red cabbage, thinly sliced
- 1 cup cucumber, julienned
- 1 cup edamame, cooked and shelled
- 1/2 cup red bell pepper, thinly sliced
- 1/4 cup green onions, sliced
- 1/4 cup cilantro, chopped
- 1/4 cup sesame seeds, toasted
- 1/4 cup slivered almonds, toasted

For the Sesame Ginger Dressing:

- 3 tablespoons soy sauce
- 2 tablespoons rice vinegar
- 1 tablespoon sesame oil
- 1 tablespoon honey or maple syrup
- 1 teaspoon grated fresh ginger
- 1 clove garlic, minced
- 1/4 cup neutral oil (vegetable or canola oil)
- Salt and black pepper to taste

Instructions:

1. In a large salad bowl, combine shredded cooked chicken, mixed salad greens, sliced red cabbage, julienned cucumber, edamame, sliced red bell pepper, green onions, and chopped cilantro.

2. In a small bowl, whisk together soy sauce, rice vinegar, sesame oil, honey or maple syrup, grated ginger, minced garlic, neutral oil, salt, and black pepper to create the dressing.

3. Pour the sesame ginger dressing over the salad and toss gently to coat the ingredients.

4. Sprinkle toasted sesame seeds and slivered almonds over the salad.

5. Serve the Asian sesame chicken salad immediately, and enjoy this flavorful and satisfying dish.

Tuna Nicoise Salad:

Ingredients:

For the Salad:

- 6 cups mixed salad greens (e.g., arugula, frisée, or butter lettuce)
- 1 pound small potatoes, boiled and halved
- 1 cup cherry tomatoes, halved
- 1 cup green beans, blanched and cut into bite-sized pieces
- 1/2 cup Nicoise olives
- 4 hard-boiled eggs, halved
- 2 (5-ounce) cans tuna, drained
- 1/4 cup red onion, thinly sliced
- Fresh parsley, chopped for garnish

For the Vinaigrette:

- 1/4 cup red wine vinegar
- 1/2 cup extra virgin olive oil
- 1 teaspoon Dijon mustard
- 1 clove garlic, minced
- Salt and black pepper to taste

Instructions:

1. In a large salad bowl, arrange mixed salad greens as the base.
2. Assemble rows of boiled and halved potatoes, cherry tomatoes, blanched green beans, Nicoise olives, hard-boiled eggs, tuna, and sliced red onion on top of the greens.
3. In a small bowl or jar, whisk together red wine vinegar, olive oil, Dijon mustard, minced garlic, salt, and black pepper to create the vinaigrette.
4. Drizzle the vinaigrette over the Tuna Nicoise salad.

5. Garnish with chopped fresh parsley.

6. Serve the Tuna Nicoise salad immediately, allowing each person to mix the ingredients and dressing according to their preference.

Watermelon Feta Salad:

Ingredients:

- 6 cups seedless watermelon, cubed
- 1 cup feta cheese, crumbled
- 1 cup cucumber, diced
- 1/4 cup fresh mint leaves, chopped
- 1/4 cup red onion, thinly sliced
- 2 tablespoons extra virgin olive oil
- 1 tablespoon balsamic glaze or balsamic reduction
- Salt and black pepper to taste

Instructions:

1. In a large salad bowl, combine cubed watermelon, crumbled feta cheese, diced cucumber, chopped fresh mint leaves, and thinly sliced red onion.

2. Drizzle extra virgin olive oil over the salad.

3. Gently toss the ingredients to combine.

4. Season the watermelon feta salad with salt and black pepper to taste.

5. Drizzle balsamic glaze or balsamic reduction over the salad for added sweetness and flavor.

6. Toss the salad once more to ensure even coating.

7. Serve the watermelon feta salad immediately as a refreshing and sweet-savory side dish.

Mexican Street Corn Salad:

Ingredients:

- 4 cups corn kernels (fresh, frozen, or canned and drained)

- 1/2 cup mayonnaise
- 1/2 cup sour cream
- 1/2 cup cotija cheese, crumbled
- 1/4 cup fresh cilantro, chopped
- 1/4 cup green onions, sliced
- 1 clove garlic, minced
- 1 teaspoon chili powder
- 1/2 teaspoon smoked paprika
- Juice of 1 lime
- Salt and black pepper to taste
- Optional: Hot sauce for extra heat

Instructions:

1. If using fresh corn, grill or cook the corn kernels until they have a slight char. If using frozen or canned corn, thaw or drain them.
2. In a large mixing bowl, combine the corn kernels, mayonnaise, sour cream, crumbled cotija cheese, chopped cilantro, sliced green onions, minced garlic, chili powder, smoked paprika, lime juice, salt, and black pepper.
3. Toss the ingredients together until well combined.
4. If desired, add hot sauce to taste for extra heat.
5. Refrigerate the Mexican street corn salad for at least 30 minutes to allow the flavors to meld.
6. Before serving, give the salad a final toss and adjust seasoning if needed.
7. Serve the Mexican street corn salad as a flavorful side dish or topping for tacos.

Orzo Pasta Salad:

Ingredients:

- 1 cup orzo pasta
- 1 cup cherry tomatoes, halved
- 1 cucumber, diced

- 1/2 red onion, finely chopped
- 1/2 cup Kalamata olives, sliced
- 1/2 cup feta cheese, crumbled
- 1/4 cup fresh parsley, chopped
- 1/4 cup extra virgin olive oil
- 2 tablespoons red wine vinegar
- 1 teaspoon Dijon mustard
- Salt and black pepper to taste
- Optional: Grilled chicken, shrimp, or chickpeas for added protein

Instructions:

1. Cook the orzo pasta according to the package instructions. Drain and let it cool.
2. In a large mixing bowl, combine the cooked and cooled orzo pasta, halved cherry tomatoes, diced cucumber, finely chopped red onion, sliced Kalamata olives, crumbled feta cheese, and chopped fresh parsley.
3. In a small bowl or jar, whisk together extra virgin olive oil, red wine vinegar, Dijon mustard, salt, and black pepper to create the dressing.
4. Pour the dressing over the orzo pasta salad and toss gently to coat all ingredients.
5. If adding protein, such as grilled chicken, shrimp, or chickpeas, incorporate them into the salad.
6. Refrigerate the orzo pasta salad for at least 30 minutes before serving to enhance the flavors.
7. Serve chilled and enjoy this refreshing and versatile orzo pasta salad.

Caesar Pasta Salad:

Ingredients:

- 8 ounces rotini or fusilli pasta, cooked and cooled
- 1 cup cherry tomatoes, halved
- 1/2 cup black olives, sliced
- 1/2 cup grated Parmesan cheese

- 1/4 cup fresh parsley, chopped
- 1/4 cup Caesar dressing
- 1 tablespoon lemon juice
- 1 teaspoon Dijon mustard
- Salt and black pepper to taste
- Optional: Grilled chicken strips for added protein

Instructions:

1. In a large mixing bowl, combine the cooked and cooled pasta, halved cherry tomatoes, sliced black olives, grated Parmesan cheese, and chopped fresh parsley.
2. In a small bowl, whisk together Caesar dressing, lemon juice, Dijon mustard, salt, and black pepper to create the dressing.
3. Pour the dressing over the pasta salad and toss gently to coat all ingredients.
4. If adding protein, such as grilled chicken strips, incorporate them into the salad.
5. Refrigerate the Caesar pasta salad for at least 30 minutes before serving to allow the flavors to meld.
6. Serve chilled and enjoy this Caesar-inspired pasta salad as a delightful and satisfying dish.

15 Dessert Recipes:

Fresh Fruit Salad:

Ingredients:

- 2 cups watermelon, cubed
- 2 cups cantaloupe, cubed
- 2 cups pineapple, cubed
- 1 cup strawberries, hulled and halved
- 1 cup grapes, halved
- 1 banana, sliced
- 1 kiwi, peeled and sliced

- 1 orange, peeled and segmented
- Fresh mint leaves for garnish (optional)

For the Citrus Honey Dressing:

- 2 tablespoons honey
- 1 tablespoon fresh orange juice
- 1 tablespoon fresh lemon juice
- Zest of 1 lemon
- Zest of 1 orange

Instructions:

1. In a large serving bowl, combine watermelon, cantaloupe, pineapple, strawberries, grapes, banana, kiwi, and orange segments.
2. In a small bowl, whisk together honey, fresh orange juice, fresh lemon juice, lemon zest, and orange zest to create the citrus honey dressing.
3. Pour the citrus honey dressing over the fresh fruit.
4. Gently toss the fruit salad to coat it evenly with the dressing.
5. Refrigerate the fresh fruit salad for at least 30 minutes before serving to enhance the flavors.
6. Before serving, garnish the fruit salad with fresh mint leaves if desired.
7. Serve chilled and enjoy this vibrant and refreshing fresh fruit salad.

Chocolate Avocado Mousse:

Ingredients:

- 2 ripe avocados, peeled and pitted
- 1/2 cup cocoa powder
- 1/2 cup maple syrup or agave syrup
- 1/4 cup almond milk or any milk of your choice
- 1 teaspoon vanilla extract
- A pinch of salt
- Optional toppings: Fresh berries, chopped nuts, shredded coconut

Instructions:

1. In a food processor or blender, combine the ripe avocados, cocoa powder, maple syrup, almond milk, vanilla extract, and a pinch of salt.
2. Blend the ingredients until smooth and creamy, scraping down the sides as needed.
3. Taste the chocolate avocado mousse and adjust sweetness if necessary by adding more maple syrup.
4. Once the mixture is smooth, transfer the chocolate avocado mousse to serving bowls or glasses.
5. Refrigerate the mousse for at least 1-2 hours to chill and allow the flavors to meld.
6. Before serving, add your choice of toppings such as fresh berries, chopped nuts, or shredded coconut.
7. Serve chilled and enjoy this decadent and healthier chocolate avocado mousse!

Baked Apples with Cinnamon:

Ingredients:

- 4 medium-sized apples (such as Granny Smith or Honeycrisp)
- 2 tablespoons unsalted butter, melted
- 2 tablespoons brown sugar
- 1 teaspoon ground cinnamon
- 1/4 teaspoon ground nutmeg
- 1/4 cup chopped nuts (walnuts or pecans), optional
- Vanilla ice cream or whipped cream for serving, optional

Instructions:

1. Preheat the oven to 375°F (190°C).
2. Wash and core the apples, leaving the bottoms intact to create a well for the filling.
3. In a small bowl, mix melted butter, brown sugar, ground cinnamon, and ground nutmeg.
4. Place the cored apples in a baking dish.

5. Spoon the cinnamon and sugar mixture into the well of each apple, distributing it evenly.

6. If using, sprinkle chopped nuts over the top of each apple.

7. Bake in the preheated oven for 25-30 minutes or until the apples are tender.

8. Remove the baked apples from the oven and let them cool slightly before serving.

9. Serve the baked apples warm, optionally with a scoop of vanilla ice cream or a dollop of whipped cream.

10. Enjoy these delicious baked apples with cinnamon as a comforting and satisfying dessert.

Chia Seed Pudding:

Ingredients:

- 1/4 cup chia seeds
- 1 cup almond milk (or any milk of your choice)
- 1 tablespoon maple syrup or honey
- 1/2 teaspoon vanilla extract
- Fresh fruit, nuts, or granola for topping (optional)

Instructions:

1. In a bowl or jar, combine chia seeds, almond milk, maple syrup or honey, and vanilla extract.

2. Stir the mixture well to ensure that the chia seeds are evenly distributed.

3. Cover the bowl or jar and refrigerate for at least 3 hours or overnight to allow the chia seeds to absorb the liquid and create a pudding-like consistency.

4. After refrigeration, give the chia pudding a good stir to break up any clumps.

5. If the pudding is too thick, you can add a little more milk to achieve your desired consistency.

6. Serve the chia seed pudding in bowls or glasses.

7. Top with fresh fruit, nuts, or granola if desired.

8. Enjoy this nutritious and customizable chia seed pudding as a healthy breakfast or snack.

Greek Yogurt Parfait:

Ingredients:

- 1 cup Greek yogurt (plain or flavored)
- 1/2 cup granola
- 1/2 cup mixed berries (strawberries, blueberries, raspberries)
- 1 tablespoon honey or maple syrup
- Optional: Nuts, seeds, or shredded coconut for garnish

Instructions:

1. In a glass or bowl, start by layering a portion of Greek yogurt at the bottom.
2. Add a layer of granola on top of the yogurt.
3. Follow with a layer of mixed berries.
4. Repeat the layers until the glass or bowl is filled.
5. Drizzle honey or maple syrup over the top for added sweetness.
6. Optionally, garnish with nuts, seeds, or shredded coconut.
7. Serve the Greek yogurt parfait immediately or refrigerate until ready to eat.
8. Enjoy this delicious and nutritious Greek yogurt parfait as a breakfast, snack, or healthy dessert.

Coconut Mango Rice Pudding:

Ingredients:

- 1 cup jasmine rice
- 2 cups coconut milk
- 1/2 cup sugar
- 1/2 teaspoon vanilla extract
- Pinch of salt
- 1 large ripe mango, peeled, pitted, and diced

- Toasted coconut flakes for garnish

Instructions:

1. Rinse the jasmine rice under cold water until the water runs clear.
2. In a medium saucepan, combine the rinsed rice, coconut milk, sugar, vanilla extract, and a pinch of salt.
3. Bring the mixture to a boil over medium heat, then reduce the heat to low, cover, and simmer for 15-20 minutes or until the rice is cooked and has absorbed the coconut milk.
4. Stir the rice occasionally to prevent sticking and ensure even cooking.
5. Once the rice is cooked and has a creamy consistency, remove the saucepan from the heat.
6. Allow the coconut mango rice pudding to cool slightly.
7. Gently fold in the diced mango.
8. Spoon the coconut mango rice pudding into serving bowls.
9. Refrigerate for at least 2 hours to chill.
10. Before serving, garnish with toasted coconut flakes.
11. Enjoy this tropical and creamy coconut mango rice pudding as a delicious dessert!

Strawberry Shortcake:

Ingredients:

For the Shortcakes:

- 2 cups all-purpose flour
- 1/4 cup granulated sugar
- 1 tablespoon baking powder
- 1/2 teaspoon salt
- 1/2 cup unsalted butter, cold and cut into small pieces
- 3/4 cup milk
- 1 teaspoon vanilla extract

For the Strawberry Filling:

- 4 cups fresh strawberries, hulled and sliced
- 1/4 cup granulated sugar (adjust based on sweetness of strawberries)
- 1 teaspoon lemon juice

For the Whipped Cream:

- 1 cup heavy cream
- 2 tablespoons powdered sugar
- 1 teaspoon vanilla extract

Instructions:

1. Preheat the oven to 425°F (220°C). Line a baking sheet with parchment paper.
2. In a large bowl, whisk together flour, sugar, baking powder, and salt.
3. Add the cold, diced butter to the flour mixture. Using a pastry cutter or your fingers, cut the butter into the flour until the mixture resembles coarse crumbs.
4. In a separate bowl, mix together milk and vanilla extract. Add the wet ingredients to the dry ingredients, stirring just until combined.
5. Turn the dough out onto a floured surface and gently knead it a few times. Pat the dough into a 1-inch thick rectangle.
6. Use a round biscuit cutter to cut out shortcakes from the dough. Place the shortcakes on the prepared baking sheet.
7. Bake for 12-15 minutes or until the tops are golden brown. Allow them to cool on a wire rack.
8. While the shortcakes are baking, prepare the strawberry filling. In a bowl, combine sliced strawberries, sugar, and lemon juice. Let the mixture sit to allow the strawberries to release their juices.
9. For the whipped cream, beat the heavy cream, powdered sugar, and vanilla extract until stiff peaks form.
10. To assemble, split the cooled shortcakes in half horizontally. Spoon the strawberry filling over the bottom half, then top with a generous dollop of whipped cream. Place the other half of the shortcake on top.
11. Serve immediately and enjoy this classic strawberry shortcake!

Lemon Sorbet:

Ingredients:

- 1 cup granulated sugar
- 1 cup water
- 1 cup fresh lemon juice (about 4-6 lemons)
- 1 tablespoon lemon zest

Instructions:

1. In a saucepan, combine granulated sugar and water. Heat over medium heat, stirring until the sugar dissolves. Bring the mixture to a gentle boil, then remove from heat.
2. Allow the sugar syrup to cool to room temperature.
3. In a bowl, combine fresh lemon juice and lemon zest.
4. Once the sugar syrup is cool, add it to the lemon juice and zest mixture. Stir well to combine.
5. Pour the lemon mixture into an ice cream maker.
6. Churn the mixture according to the manufacturer's instructions until it reaches a sorbet consistency.
7. Transfer the lemon sorbet to a lidded container and freeze for an additional 2-3 hours to firm up.
8. Before serving, let the sorbet soften for a few minutes at room temperature.
9. Scoop the lemon sorbet into bowls or cones, and enjoy this refreshing and tangy frozen treat!

Banana Ice Cream:

Ingredients:

- 4 ripe bananas, peeled, sliced, and frozen
- 1 teaspoon vanilla extract (optional)
- Toppings of your choice: chopped nuts, chocolate chips, or honey (optional)

Instructions:

1. Peel ripe bananas, slice them into rounds, and place the slices in a single layer on a parchment paper-lined tray or plate.

2. Freeze the banana slices for at least 2 hours or until solid.

3. Once frozen, transfer the banana slices to a blender or food processor.

4. Add vanilla extract, if using.

5. Blend the frozen banana slices until smooth and creamy. You may need to stop and scrape down the sides occasionally.

6. The mixture will resemble soft-serve ice cream. If you prefer a firmer texture, transfer the banana ice cream to a lidded container and freeze for an additional 1-2 hours.

7. Before serving, let the banana ice cream soften for a few minutes at room temperature.

8. Scoop the banana ice cream into bowls or cones.

9. Optional: Add your favorite toppings such as chopped nuts, chocolate chips, or a drizzle of honey.

10. Enjoy this simple and healthy banana ice cream as a guilt-free frozen treat!

Berry Yogurt Popsicles:

Ingredients:

- 1 cup mixed berries (strawberries, blueberries, raspberries)
- 1 cup Greek yogurt (plain or flavored)
- 2 tablespoons honey or maple syrup
- 1/2 teaspoon vanilla extract (optional)

Instructions:

1. In a blender, combine mixed berries, Greek yogurt, honey or maple syrup, and vanilla extract.

2. Blend the ingredients until smooth.

3. Taste the mixture and adjust sweetness if needed by adding more honey or maple syrup.

4. Pour the berry yogurt mixture into popsicle molds, leaving a little space at the top for expansion.

5. Insert popsicle sticks into the molds.

6. Freeze the popsicles for at least 4-6 hours or until completely frozen.

7. Once frozen, run the popsicle molds under warm water for a few seconds to help release the popsicles.

8. Remove the berry yogurt popsicles from the molds and serve immediately.

9. Enjoy these refreshing and healthy popsicles as a cool treat on a hot day!

Peach Cobbler:

Ingredients:

For the Peach Filling:

- 6 cups fresh peaches, peeled and sliced
- 1/2 cup granulated sugar
- 1 tablespoon lemon juice
- 1 teaspoon vanilla extract
- 2 tablespoons cornstarch

For the Cobbler Topping:

- 1 cup all-purpose flour
- 1/2 cup granulated sugar
- 1 teaspoon baking powder
- 1/4 teaspoon salt
- 1/2 cup unsalted butter, melted
- 1/4 cup boiling water

For Serving:

- Vanilla ice cream or whipped cream (optional)

Instructions:

1. Preheat the oven to 375°F (190°C).

2. In a large mixing bowl, combine sliced peaches, granulated sugar, lemon juice, vanilla extract, and cornstarch. Toss until the peaches are evenly coated.

3. Transfer the peach filling to a 9x13-inch baking dish, spreading it evenly.

4. In a separate bowl, whisk together flour, sugar, baking powder, and salt for the cobbler topping.

5. Add melted butter to the flour mixture and stir until just combined.

6. Gradually add boiling water to the cobbler batter, mixing until smooth.

7. Spoon the cobbler batter over the peach filling in the baking dish, spreading it evenly.

8. Bake in the preheated oven for 40-45 minutes or until the cobbler topping is golden brown and the peach filling is bubbly.

9. Allow the peach cobbler to cool for a few minutes before serving.

10. Serve warm, optionally with a scoop of vanilla ice cream or a dollop of whipped cream.

11. Enjoy this classic peach cobbler as a comforting and delicious dessert!

Dark Chocolate-Dipped Strawberries:

Ingredients:

- Fresh strawberries, washed and dried
- 6 ounces dark chocolate, finely chopped
- 1 tablespoon coconut oil or vegetable shortening (optional, for smoother consistency)
- Toppings of your choice: chopped nuts, shredded coconut, sprinkles (optional)

Instructions:

1. Line a baking sheet with parchment paper.

2. In a heatproof bowl, melt the dark chocolate using one of the following methods:
   - Microwave: Heat in 20-second intervals, stirring between each interval until smooth.

- Double Boiler: Place the bowl over a pot of simmering water, stirring until melted.

3. If desired, add coconut oil or vegetable shortening to the melted chocolate and stir until well combined. This helps create a smoother consistency for dipping.

4. Hold each strawberry by the stem and dip it into the melted chocolate, ensuring the strawberry is well-coated.

5. Allow excess chocolate to drip off, then place the dipped strawberry on the prepared baking sheet.

6. If using toppings, sprinkle them onto the chocolate-covered strawberries before the chocolate sets.

7. Repeat the dipping process for each strawberry.

8. Place the baking sheet in the refrigerator for about 30 minutes or until the chocolate has set.

9. Once set, transfer the dark chocolate-dipped strawberries to a serving plate.

Pumpkin Pie Smoothie:

Ingredients:

- 1/2 cup canned pumpkin puree
- 1 ripe banana, frozen
- 1/2 cup vanilla yogurt
- 1/2 cup milk (dairy or plant-based)
- 1/2 teaspoon pumpkin pie spice
- 1 tablespoon maple syrup or honey (optional, for sweetness)
- Ice cubes (optional)

Instructions:

1. In a blender, combine canned pumpkin puree, frozen banana, vanilla yogurt, milk, pumpkin pie spice, and maple syrup or honey.

2. Blend until smooth and creamy. If the smoothie is too thick, you can add more milk to achieve your desired consistency.

3. Taste the smoothie and adjust sweetness if needed by adding more maple syrup or honey.

4. If a colder smoothie is desired, add ice cubes and blend until smooth.

5. Pour the pumpkin pie smoothie into a glass.

6. Optionally, garnish with a sprinkle of pumpkin pie spice on top.

7. Serve immediately and enjoy this seasonal and flavorful pumpkin pie smoothie!

Almond Flour Blueberry Muffins:

Ingredients:

- 2 cups almond flour
- 1/4 cup coconut flour
- 1/2 teaspoon baking soda
- 1/4 teaspoon salt
- 3 large eggs
- 1/4 cup melted coconut oil or melted butter
- 1/3 cup honey or maple syrup
- 1 teaspoon vanilla extract
- 1 cup fresh or frozen blueberries

Instructions:

1. Preheat the oven to 350°F (175°C). Line a muffin tin with paper liners or grease the cups.

2. In a large bowl, whisk together almond flour, coconut flour, baking soda, and salt.

3. In a separate bowl, beat the eggs. Add melted coconut oil or butter, honey or maple syrup, and vanilla extract. Mix well.

4. Pour the wet ingredients into the dry ingredients and stir until just combined.

5. Gently fold in the blueberries.

6. Spoon the batter into the muffin cups, filling each about 3/4 full.

7. Bake in the preheated oven for 18-22 minutes or until a toothpick inserted into the center comes out clean.

8. Allow the muffins to cool in the tin for 5 minutes, then transfer them to a wire rack to cool completely.

9. Once cooled, serve and enjoy these almond flour blueberry muffins as a gluten-free and delicious treat!

Caramelized Pineapple with Coconut:

Ingredients:

- 1 pineapple, peeled, cored, and cut into bite-sized chunks
- 1/4 cup brown sugar
- 2 tablespoons unsweetened shredded coconut
- 2 tablespoons unsalted butter
- Pinch of salt

Instructions:

1. In a large skillet over medium heat, melt the butter.

2. Add the pineapple chunks to the skillet and sprinkle brown sugar over them.

3. Stir the pineapple to coat it evenly with the melted butter and sugar.

4. Cook the pineapple for 8-10 minutes, stirring occasionally, until it becomes golden brown and caramelized.

5. Add shredded coconut to the skillet and continue cooking for an additional 2-3 minutes, allowing the coconut to toast and enhance its flavor.

6. Sprinkle a pinch of salt over the caramelized pineapple and coconut mixture. Stir to combine.

7. Once the pineapple is caramelized to your liking and the coconut is toasted, remove the skillet from the heat.

8. Transfer the caramelized pineapple with coconut to a serving dish.

9. Serve warm as a delicious dessert, snack, or topping for yogurt or ice cream.

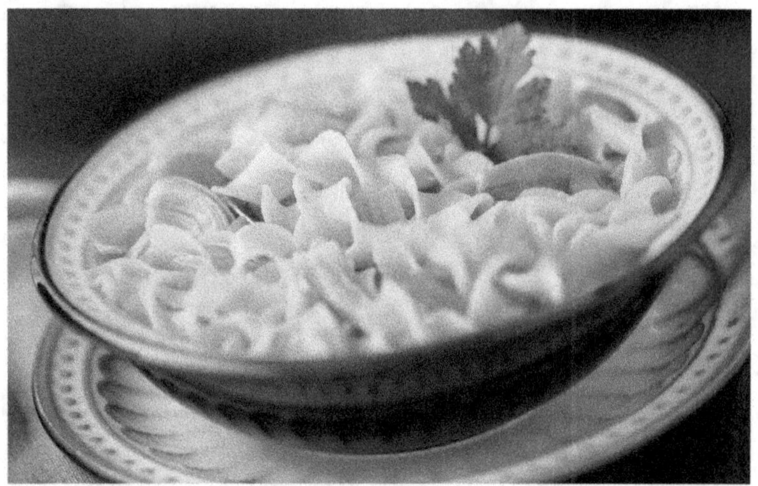

Chicken Noodle Soup:

Ingredients:

- 1 tablespoon olive oil
- 1 onion, diced
- 2 carrots, sliced
- 2 celery stalks, sliced
- 3 cloves garlic, minced
- 6 cups chicken broth
- 1 bay leaf
- 1 teaspoon dried thyme
- 1 teaspoon dried oregano
- 1 teaspoon salt, or to taste
- 1/2 teaspoon black pepper, or to taste

- 2 cups cooked chicken, shredded or diced
- 2 cups egg noodles
- 1/4 cup fresh parsley, chopped
- Lemon wedges for serving (optional)

Instructions:

1. In a large pot, heat olive oil over medium heat. Add diced onion, sliced carrots, sliced celery, and minced garlic. Sauté for 5-7 minutes until vegetables are softened.

2. Pour in chicken broth and add the bay leaf, dried thyme, dried oregano, salt, and black pepper. Bring the mixture to a simmer.

3. Add the cooked chicken to the pot and continue simmering for an additional 10 minutes.

4. Add the egg noodles to the pot and cook according to package instructions until they are tender.

5. Once the noodles are cooked, remove the bay leaf from the soup.

6. Stir in chopped fresh parsley.

7. Taste the soup and adjust salt and pepper if needed.

8. Serve the chicken noodle soup hot, optionally with lemon wedges on the side for a burst of citrus flavor.

9. Enjoy this comforting and classic chicken noodle soup as a satisfying meal.

Minestrone Soup:

Ingredients:

- 2 tablespoons olive oil
- 1 onion, diced
- 2 carrots, diced
- 2 celery stalks, diced
- 3 cloves garlic, minced
- 1 zucchini, diced

- 1 yellow squash, diced
- 1 teaspoon dried oregano
- 1 teaspoon dried basil
- 1/2 teaspoon dried thyme
- 1 can (14 oz) diced tomatoes, undrained
- 1 can (15 oz) kidney beans, drained and rinsed
- 6 cups vegetable broth
- 1 cup small pasta (such as ditalini or elbow macaroni)
- Salt and black pepper to taste
- 2 cups fresh spinach, chopped
- Grated Parmesan cheese for serving (optional)

Instructions:

1. In a large pot, heat olive oil over medium heat. Add diced onion, carrots, celery, and minced garlic. Sauté for 5-7 minutes until vegetables are softened.
2. Add diced zucchini and yellow squash to the pot. Continue to cook for an additional 5 minutes.
3. Stir in dried oregano, dried basil, and dried thyme. Cook for 1-2 minutes to allow the herbs to become fragrant.
4. Pour in diced tomatoes with their juice, kidney beans, and vegetable broth. Bring the mixture to a boil.
5. Add the small pasta to the pot and cook according to package instructions until al dente.
6. Season the minestrone soup with salt and black pepper to taste.
7. Just before serving, stir in chopped fresh spinach and cook until wilted.
8. Taste and adjust the seasoning if needed.
9. Serve the minestrone soup hot, optionally topped with grated Parmesan cheese.
10. Enjoy this hearty and flavorful minestrone soup as a wholesome and satisfying meal.

Tomato Basil Soup:

Ingredients:

- 2 tablespoons olive oil
- 1 onion, chopped
- 3 cloves garlic, minced
- 2 cans (28 oz each) whole tomatoes, undrained
- 1/4 cup tomato paste
- 2 cups vegetable broth
- 1 teaspoon sugar
- 1 teaspoon dried basil
- 1/2 teaspoon dried oregano
- Salt and black pepper to taste
- 1/2 cup heavy cream (optional, for a creamy version)
- Fresh basil leaves for garnish (optional)

Instructions:

1. In a large pot, heat olive oil over medium heat. Add chopped onion and sauté until softened, about 5 minutes.
2. Add minced garlic to the pot and sauté for an additional 1-2 minutes until fragrant.
3. Pour in the whole tomatoes with their juice. Break up the tomatoes using a spoon or spatula.
4. Stir in tomato paste, vegetable broth, sugar, dried basil, dried oregano, salt, and black pepper.
5. Bring the mixture to a simmer and let it cook for 15-20 minutes, allowing the flavors to meld.
6. If you prefer a creamy tomato basil soup, stir in the heavy cream at this stage.
7. Use an immersion blender to puree the soup until smooth. Alternatively, transfer the soup in batches to a blender and blend until smooth, then return it to the pot.
8. Taste the soup and adjust the seasoning if needed.
9. Serve the tomato basil soup hot, optionally garnished with fresh basil leaves.

10. Enjoy this classic and comforting tomato basil soup on its own or with a side of crusty bread.

Lentil Soup:

Ingredients:

- 1 cup dried green or brown lentils, rinsed and drained
- 2 tablespoons olive oil
- 1 onion, chopped
- 2 carrots, diced
- 2 celery stalks, diced
- 3 cloves garlic, minced
- 1 teaspoon ground cumin
- 1 teaspoon ground coriander
- 1 teaspoon paprika
- 1/2 teaspoon turmeric
- 6 cups vegetable or chicken broth
- 1 can (14 oz) diced tomatoes, undrained
- 1 bay leaf
- Salt and black pepper to taste
- Juice of 1 lemon (optional, for serving)
- Fresh parsley for garnish (optional)

Instructions:

1. In a large pot, heat olive oil over medium heat. Add chopped onion, diced carrots, and diced celery. Sauté for 5-7 minutes until vegetables are softened.
2. Add minced garlic to the pot and cook for an additional 1-2 minutes until fragrant.
3. Stir in ground cumin, ground coriander, paprika, and turmeric. Cook for 1-2 minutes to toast the spices.
4. Pour in rinsed lentils, vegetable or chicken broth, diced tomatoes with their juice, and add the bay leaf. Bring the mixture to a boil.

5. Reduce the heat to low, cover the pot, and simmer for 25-30 minutes or until the lentils are tender.

6. Season the lentil soup with salt and black pepper to taste.

7. Just before serving, squeeze the juice of one lemon into the soup for a burst of freshness if desired.

8. Remove the bay leaf from the soup.

9. Ladle the lentil soup into bowls and garnish with fresh parsley if desired.

10. Serve the lentil soup hot and enjoy this wholesome and nutritious dish.

Butternut Squash Soup:

Ingredients:

- 1 large butternut squash, peeled, seeded, and diced
- 2 tablespoons olive oil
- 1 onion, chopped
- 2 carrots, chopped
- 2 celery stalks, chopped
- 3 cloves garlic, minced
- 1 teaspoon ground cumin
- 1/2 teaspoon ground cinnamon
- 1/4 teaspoon ground nutmeg
- 6 cups vegetable or chicken broth
- Salt and black pepper to taste
- 1/2 cup heavy cream or coconut milk (optional, for creaminess)
- Toasted pumpkin seeds for garnish (optional)
- Fresh parsley or chives for garnish (optional)

Instructions:

1. Preheat the oven to 400°F (200°C).

2. Place the diced butternut squash on a baking sheet. Drizzle with 1 tablespoon of olive oil and toss to coat. Roast in the preheated oven for 25-30 minutes or until the squash is tender and lightly caramelized.

3. In a large pot, heat the remaining 1 tablespoon of olive oil over medium heat. Add chopped onion, carrots, and celery. Sauté for 5-7 minutes until the vegetables are softened.

4. Add minced garlic to the pot and cook for an additional 1-2 minutes until fragrant.

5. Stir in ground cumin, ground cinnamon, and ground nutmeg. Cook for 1-2 minutes to toast the spices.

6. Add the roasted butternut squash to the pot and pour in vegetable or chicken broth. Bring the mixture to a simmer.

7. Use an immersion blender to puree the soup until smooth. Alternatively, transfer the soup in batches to a blender and blend until smooth, then return it to the pot.

8. Season the butternut squash soup with salt and black pepper to taste.

9. If you prefer a creamy texture, stir in heavy cream or coconut milk.

10. Heat the soup through but avoid boiling once the cream or coconut milk is added.

11. Taste and adjust the seasoning if needed.

12. Serve the butternut squash soup hot, optionally garnished with toasted pumpkin seeds, fresh parsley, or chives.

Vegetarian Chili:

Ingredients:

- 2 tablespoons olive oil
- 1 large onion, diced
- 3 cloves garlic, minced
- 1 bell pepper, diced (any color)
- 1 zucchini, diced
- 1 carrot, diced
- 1 celery stalk, diced

- 2 cans (15 oz each) black beans, drained and rinsed
- 2 cans (15 oz each) kidney beans, drained and rinsed
- 1 can (28 oz) crushed tomatoes
- 1 can (14 oz) diced tomatoes with green chilies
- 2 cups vegetable broth
- 2 teaspoons ground cumin
- 2 teaspoons chili powder
- 1 teaspoon paprika
- 1/2 teaspoon dried oregano
- Salt and black pepper to taste
- 1 cup frozen corn kernels
- Juice of 1 lime (optional, for serving)
- Fresh cilantro for garnish (optional)
- Shredded cheese, sour cream, or avocado slices for toppings (optional)

Instructions:

1. In a large pot, heat olive oil over medium heat. Add diced onion, minced garlic, diced bell pepper, diced zucchini, diced carrot, and diced celery. Sauté for 5-7 minutes until vegetables are softened.

2. Add drained black beans, drained kidney beans, crushed tomatoes, diced tomatoes with green chilies, and vegetable broth to the pot.

3. Stir in ground cumin, chili powder, paprika, dried oregano, salt, and black pepper. Mix well.

4. Bring the chili to a simmer, then reduce the heat to low, cover the pot, and let it simmer for at least 30 minutes to allow the flavors to meld.

5. Add frozen corn kernels to the chili and simmer for an additional 10 minutes.

6. Taste the chili and adjust the seasoning if needed.

7. Just before serving, stir in the lime juice if using.

8. Ladle the vegetarian chili into bowls and garnish with fresh cilantro if desired.

9. Optionally, serve the chili with shredded cheese, a dollop of sour cream, or slices of avocado.

10. Enjoy this hearty and flavorful vegetarian chili as a satisfying and wholesome meal.

Broccoli Cheddar Soup:

Ingredients:

- 1/4 cup unsalted butter
- 1 onion, diced
- 2 carrots, peeled and diced
- 2 celery stalks, diced
- 3 cloves garlic, minced
- 1/4 cup all-purpose flour
- 3 cups vegetable or chicken broth
- 3 cups broccoli florets
- 2 cups shredded sharp cheddar cheese
- 2 cups milk (whole or 2%)
- Salt and black pepper to taste
- 1/2 teaspoon dried thyme
- 1/2 teaspoon paprika
- 1/4 teaspoon ground nutmeg
- Optional: Additional shredded cheddar cheese for garnish

Instructions:

1. In a large pot, melt the butter over medium heat. Add diced onion, diced carrots, diced celery, and minced garlic. Sauté for 5-7 minutes until the vegetables are softened.

2. Sprinkle flour over the sautéed vegetables and stir to coat. Cook for an additional 1-2 minutes to remove the raw taste of the flour.

3. Gradually whisk in vegetable or chicken broth, ensuring there are no lumps.

4. Add broccoli florets to the pot and simmer for 15-20 minutes or until the broccoli is tender.

5. Use an immersion blender to puree the soup until smooth. Alternatively, transfer the soup in batches to a blender and blend until smooth, then return it to the pot.

6. Stir in shredded sharp cheddar cheese until melted and incorporated into the soup.

7. Pour in milk and continue to cook over medium heat, stirring occasionally, until the soup is heated through.

8. Season the soup with salt, black pepper, dried thyme, paprika, and ground nutmeg. Adjust the seasoning to your liking.

9. Optionally, garnish the broccoli cheddar soup with additional shredded cheddar cheese just before serving.

10. Serve the soup hot and enjoy this creamy and comforting broccoli cheddar soup!

Chicken Tortilla Soup:

Ingredients:

- 1 tablespoon olive oil
- 1 onion, diced
- 2 cloves garlic, minced
- 1 jalapeño, seeds and ribs removed, minced
- 1 teaspoon ground cumin
- 1 teaspoon chili powder
- 1/2 teaspoon paprika
- 1 can (14 oz) diced tomatoes with green chilies
- 1 can (15 oz) black beans, drained and rinsed
- 1 cup corn kernels (fresh or frozen)
- 1 red bell pepper, diced
- 1 zucchini, diced
- 6 cups chicken broth
- 2 cups cooked chicken, shredded

- Salt and black pepper to taste
- Juice of 1 lime
- Fresh cilantro for garnish
- Tortilla strips or chips for serving
- Avocado slices for serving
- Shredded cheese for serving (optional)
- Sour cream for serving (optional)

Instructions:

1. In a large pot, heat olive oil over medium heat. Add diced onion, minced garlic, and minced jalapeño. Sauté for 3-4 minutes until the vegetables are softened.
2. Stir in ground cumin, chili powder, and paprika. Cook for an additional 1-2 minutes to toast the spices.
3. Add diced tomatoes with green chilies, black beans, corn kernels, diced red bell pepper, and diced zucchini to the pot. Mix well.
4. Pour in chicken broth and bring the mixture to a boil.
5. Reduce the heat to low, add shredded chicken to the pot, and simmer for 15-20 minutes to allow the flavors to meld.
6. Season the chicken tortilla soup with salt and black pepper to taste.
7. Just before serving, stir in the lime juice.
8. Ladle the soup into bowls and garnish with fresh cilantro.
9. Optionally, serve the chicken tortilla soup with tortilla strips or chips, avocado slices, shredded cheese, and sour cream.
10. Enjoy this flavorful and hearty chicken tortilla soup as a satisfying and comforting meal.

Split Pea Soup:

Ingredients:

- 1 tablespoon olive oil
- 1 onion, chopped

- 2 carrots, diced
- 2 celery stalks, diced
- 3 cloves garlic, minced
- 1 pound (about 2 cups) dried green split peas, rinsed and drained
- 8 cups vegetable or ham broth
- 1 bay leaf
- 1 teaspoon dried thyme
- 1 teaspoon dried oregano
- Salt and black pepper to taste
- 1 cup diced ham (optional)
- 1 cup diced potatoes (optional)
- 1 cup diced ham (optional)
- Fresh parsley for garnish (optional)

Instructions:

1. In a large pot, heat olive oil over medium heat. Add chopped onion, diced carrots, and diced celery. Sauté for 5-7 minutes until the vegetables are softened.
2. Add minced garlic to the pot and cook for an additional 1-2 minutes until fragrant.
3. Stir in dried green split peas, vegetable or ham broth, bay leaf, dried thyme, dried oregano, salt, and black pepper.
4. Bring the soup to a boil, then reduce the heat to low and cover the pot.
5. Simmer the split pea soup for 1 to 1.5 hours, stirring occasionally, until the split peas are tender and the soup has thickened.
6. If using, add diced ham and diced potatoes to the pot and continue simmering for an additional 30 minutes or until the potatoes are cooked through.
7. Taste the split pea soup and adjust the seasoning if needed.
8. Remove the bay leaf from the soup.
9. Optionally, use an immersion blender to puree the soup partially for a creamier texture while leaving some split peas intact.
10. Ladle the split pea soup into bowls and garnish with fresh parsley if desired.

11. Enjoy this hearty and comforting split pea soup as a satisfying and nutritious meal.

Thai Coconut Soup (Tom Kha Gai):

Ingredients:

- 1 tablespoon vegetable oil
- 1 onion, thinly sliced
- 2 cloves garlic, minced
- 1 tablespoon fresh ginger, grated
- 2 tablespoons Thai red curry paste
- 3 cups chicken or vegetable broth
- 1 can (14 oz) coconut milk
- 1 tablespoon soy sauce
- 1 tablespoon fish sauce (omit for vegetarian version)
- 1 tablespoon brown sugar
- 1 stalk lemongrass, cut into 3-inch pieces and bruised
- 2 kaffir lime leaves (optional)
- 8 ounces mushrooms, sliced
- 1 pound boneless, skinless chicken thighs, thinly sliced (optional for chicken version)
- 1 medium-sized tomato, diced
- Juice of 1 lime
- Fresh cilantro leaves for garnish
- Thai bird chilies or red pepper flakes for heat (optional)

Instructions:

1. In a large pot, heat vegetable oil over medium heat. Add thinly sliced onion, minced garlic, and grated ginger. Sauté for 2-3 minutes until the onions are softened.
2. Stir in Thai red curry paste and cook for an additional 1-2 minutes until fragrant.

3. Pour in chicken or vegetable broth, coconut milk, soy sauce, fish sauce, and brown sugar. Mix well.

4. Add bruised lemongrass, kaffir lime leaves (if using), sliced mushrooms, and sliced chicken thighs (if using). Bring the soup to a gentle simmer.

5. Simmer the soup for 15-20 minutes, allowing the flavors to meld.

6. Add diced tomatoes to the soup and cook for an additional 5 minutes.

7. Stir in lime juice to brighten the flavors.

8. Taste the Thai coconut soup and adjust the seasoning, adding more soy sauce, fish sauce, or lime juice if needed. For additional heat, add Thai bird chilies or red pepper flakes.

9. Remove lemongrass stalks and kaffir lime leaves from the soup.

10. Ladle the Thai coconut soup into bowls, garnish with fresh cilantro leaves, and serve hot.

11. Enjoy this aromatic and flavorful Tom Kha Gai as a comforting and exotic soup.

Vegetable Barley Soup:

Ingredients:

- 1 tablespoon olive oil
- 1 onion, diced
- 2 carrots, diced
- 2 celery stalks, diced
- 3 cloves garlic, minced
- 1 cup pearl barley, rinsed and drained
- 8 cups vegetable broth
- 1 can (14 oz) diced tomatoes
- 2 bay leaves
- 1 teaspoon dried thyme
- 1 teaspoon dried rosemary
- Salt and black pepper to taste

- 2 cups chopped seasonal vegetables (e.g., green beans, zucchini, bell peppers)
- 1 cup spinach or kale, chopped
- Fresh parsley for garnish

Instructions:

1. In a large pot, heat olive oil over medium heat. Add diced onion, diced carrots, and diced celery. Sauté for 5-7 minutes until the vegetables are softened.
2. Add minced garlic to the pot and cook for an additional 1-2 minutes until fragrant.
3. Stir in pearl barley and cook for 1-2 minutes to lightly toast the barley.
4. Pour in vegetable broth, diced tomatoes, bay leaves, dried thyme, dried rosemary, salt, and black pepper. Mix well.
5. Bring the vegetable barley soup to a boil, then reduce the heat to low and cover the pot.
6. Simmer the soup for 30-40 minutes or until the barley is tender.
7. Add chopped seasonal vegetables to the pot and continue simmering for an additional 10-15 minutes until the vegetables are cooked to your liking.
8. Stir in chopped spinach or kale and cook for an additional 2-3 minutes until wilted.
9. Taste the soup and adjust the seasoning if needed.
10. Remove the bay leaves from the soup.
11. Ladle the vegetable barley soup into bowls, garnish with fresh parsley, and serve hot.

French Onion Soup:

Ingredients:

- 4 large onions, thinly sliced
- 3 tablespoons butter
- 2 tablespoons olive oil
- 1 teaspoon sugar
- 2 cloves garlic, minced

- 1/2 cup dry white wine (optional)
- 6 cups beef broth
- 2 bay leaves
- 1 teaspoon dried thyme
- Salt and black pepper to taste
- Baguette slices
- 2 cups grated Gruyère or Swiss cheese

Instructions:

1. In a large pot, melt butter and olive oil over medium heat. Add thinly sliced onions and cook for about 15-20 minutes, stirring occasionally, until the onions are soft and caramelized.
2. Sprinkle sugar over the onions and continue cooking for an additional 5 minutes to enhance caramelization.
3. Add minced garlic to the pot and cook for 1-2 minutes until fragrant.
4. If using, pour in the dry white wine to deglaze the pot, scraping up any brown bits from the bottom.
5. Pour in beef broth, add bay leaves, dried thyme, salt, and black pepper. Bring the soup to a simmer and let it cook for an additional 15-20 minutes to allow the flavors to meld.
6. Meanwhile, preheat the broiler.
7. Arrange baguette slices on a baking sheet and toast them under the broiler for 1-2 minutes on each side until golden brown.
8. Remove bay leaves from the soup and discard them.
9. Ladle the French onion soup into oven-safe bowls.
10. Place a couple of toasted baguette slices on top of the soup in each bowl.
11. Sprinkle a generous amount of grated Gruyère or Swiss cheese over the baguette slices.
12. Place the bowls under the broiler for 2-3 minutes, or until the cheese is melted and bubbly, with a golden-brown crust.

13. Carefully remove the bowls from the broiler, and let them cool slightly before serving.

14. Enjoy this classic French onion soup with its rich, flavorful broth and gooey melted cheese.

Miso Soup:

Ingredients:

- 4 cups dashi (Japanese broth, can be made with kombu and bonito flakes)
- 3 tablespoons miso paste (white or red miso)
- 1 cup firm tofu, cubed
- 2 green onions, thinly sliced
- 1 sheet nori (seaweed), cut into thin strips (optional)
- 1 cup mushrooms, sliced (shiitake or enoki work well)
- 1 cup spinach or baby bok choy, chopped
- Soy sauce to taste (optional)
- Sesame oil for drizzling (optional)

Instructions:

1. In a pot, heat the dashi over medium heat. Bring it to a gentle simmer but avoid boiling.

2. While the dashi is heating, dissolve miso paste in a small bowl with a ladleful of the hot dashi. Whisk until the miso paste is fully incorporated.

3. Add the miso mixture back into the pot with the remaining dashi, stirring well to combine.

4. Add cubed tofu, sliced green onions, nori strips (if using), mushrooms, and spinach or baby bok choy to the pot. Let it simmer for a few minutes until the vegetables are tender.

5. Taste the miso soup and adjust the flavor with soy sauce if needed. Be cautious with the saltiness, as miso is already salty.

6. Once the ingredients are cooked to your liking, remove the pot from heat.

7. Ladle the miso soup into bowls, and drizzle with a bit of sesame oil if desired.

8. Serve the miso soup hot and enjoy this traditional Japanese comfort food.

Roasted Red Pepper Soup:

Ingredients:

- 4 red bell peppers, halved and seeds removed
- 2 tablespoons olive oil
- 1 onion, chopped
- 2 carrots, chopped
- 2 celery stalks, chopped
- 3 cloves garlic, minced
- 4 cups vegetable broth
- 1 can (14 oz) diced tomatoes
- 1 teaspoon dried basil
- 1 teaspoon dried oregano
- 1/2 teaspoon smoked paprika
- Salt and black pepper to taste
- 1/2 cup heavy cream or coconut milk (optional, for creaminess)
- Fresh basil leaves for garnish (optional)

Instructions:

1. Preheat the oven to 400°F (200°C).

2. Place red bell pepper halves, cut side down, on a baking sheet. Roast in the preheated oven for 25-30 minutes or until the peppers' skins are charred and blistered.

3. Once roasted, transfer the peppers to a bowl, cover with plastic wrap, and let them steam for 10 minutes. This will make it easier to peel off the skin.

4. While the peppers are steaming, heat olive oil in a large pot over medium heat. Add chopped onion, chopped carrots, and chopped celery. Sauté for 5-7 minutes until the vegetables are softened.

5. Add minced garlic to the pot and cook for an additional 1-2 minutes until fragrant.

6. Peel the skins off the roasted red peppers and chop them. Add the chopped peppers to the pot.

7. Pour in vegetable broth, diced tomatoes with their juice, dried basil, dried oregano, smoked paprika, salt, and black pepper. Bring the mixture to a boil, then reduce the heat to low, cover the pot, and simmer for 20-25 minutes.

8. Use an immersion blender to puree the soup until smooth. Alternatively, transfer the soup in batches to a blender and blend until smooth, then return it to the pot.

9. If you prefer a creamy texture, stir in heavy cream or coconut milk.

10. Heat the soup through but avoid boiling once the cream or coconut milk is added.

11. Taste the soup and adjust the seasoning if needed.

12. Ladle the roasted red pepper soup into bowls, garnish with fresh basil leaves if desired, and serve hot.

Cauliflower Soup:

Ingredients:

- 1 large cauliflower, chopped into florets
- 2 tablespoons olive oil
- 1 onion, chopped
- 2 cloves garlic, minced
- 1 potato, peeled and diced
- 4 cups vegetable broth
- 1 teaspoon ground cumin
- 1/2 teaspoon ground coriander
- 1/2 teaspoon dried thyme
- Salt and black pepper to taste
- 1 cup milk or plant-based milk
- 1/4 cup grated Parmesan cheese or nutritional yeast (optional, for added flavor)
- Fresh chives or parsley for garnish (optional)

Instructions:

1. Preheat the oven to 400°F (200°C).

2. Toss cauliflower florets with olive oil on a baking sheet. Roast in the preheated oven for 25-30 minutes or until the cauliflower is golden brown and tender.

3. In a large pot, heat olive oil over medium heat. Add chopped onion and cook for 5-7 minutes until softened.

4. Add minced garlic to the pot and cook for an additional 1-2 minutes until fragrant.

5. Stir in diced potato, roasted cauliflower, vegetable broth, ground cumin, ground coriander, dried thyme, salt, and black pepper. Bring the mixture to a boil, then reduce the heat to low, cover the pot, and simmer for 15-20 minutes until the potatoes are cooked through.

6. Use an immersion blender to puree the soup until smooth. Alternatively, transfer the soup in batches to a blender and blend until smooth, then return it to the pot.

7. Stir in milk and continue to cook over medium heat, stirring occasionally, until the soup is heated through.

8. If using, add grated Parmesan cheese or nutritional yeast for added flavor. Stir until the cheese is melted and incorporated into the soup.

9. Taste the cauliflower soup and adjust the seasoning if needed.

10. Ladle the soup into bowls, garnish with fresh chives or parsley if desired, and serve hot.

Stew Recipes:

Beef Stew:

Ingredients:

- 2 pounds stewing beef, cut into cubes
- 1/4 cup all-purpose flour
- Salt and black pepper to taste
- 2 tablespoons vegetable oil

- 1 onion, chopped
- 3 cloves garlic, minced
- 4 cups beef broth
- 1 cup red wine (optional)
- 2 tablespoons tomato paste
- 1 teaspoon dried thyme
- 2 bay leaves
- 4 carrots, peeled and sliced
- 3 potatoes, peeled and diced
- 1 cup frozen peas (optional)
- Fresh parsley for garnish

Instructions:

1. In a bowl, combine the cubed stewing beef with flour, salt, and black pepper. Toss to coat the beef evenly.
2. In a large pot, heat vegetable oil over medium-high heat. Add the coated beef cubes and brown them on all sides. Work in batches to avoid overcrowding the pot. Remove the browned beef from the pot and set it aside.
3. In the same pot, add chopped onion and minced garlic. Sauté for 5-7 minutes until the onion is softened.
4. Pour in beef broth and red wine (if using), scraping up any brown bits from the bottom of the pot for added flavor.
5. Stir in tomato paste, dried thyme, and add bay leaves. Return the browned beef to the pot and bring the mixture to a simmer.
6. Cover the pot and let the beef stew simmer on low heat for about 1.5 to 2 hours, or until the beef is tender.
7. Add sliced carrots and diced potatoes to the pot. Continue simmering for an additional 30-45 minutes until the vegetables are cooked through.
8. If using, add frozen peas to the pot and cook for an additional 5 minutes until heated through.

9. Taste the beef stew and adjust the seasoning if needed. Remove bay leaves.

10. Ladle the beef stew into bowls, garnish with fresh parsley, and serve hot.

Chicken and Dumplings:

Ingredients:

For the Chicken Stew:

- 1 whole chicken (about 4 pounds), cut into pieces
- 2 tablespoons vegetable oil
- 1 onion, chopped
- 3 carrots, sliced
- 3 celery stalks, sliced
- 4 cups chicken broth
- 1 teaspoon dried thyme
- Salt and black pepper to taste
- 1 cup frozen peas
- 1/2 cup heavy cream (optional)
- Fresh parsley for garnish

For the Dumplings:

- 2 cups all-purpose flour
- 1 tablespoon baking powder
- 1 teaspoon salt
- 1 cup milk
- 1/2 cup unsalted butter, melted

Instructions:

For the Chicken Stew:

1. In a large pot, heat vegetable oil over medium-high heat. Brown the chicken pieces on all sides. Remove the chicken from the pot and set aside.

2. In the same pot, add chopped onion, sliced carrots, and sliced celery. Sauté for 5-7 minutes until the vegetables are softened.

3. Return the browned chicken to the pot. Pour in chicken broth, add dried thyme, salt, and black pepper. Bring the mixture to a simmer.

4. Cover the pot and let the chicken stew simmer for 45-60 minutes or until the chicken is cooked through and tender.

5. Remove the chicken from the pot. Once cool enough to handle, shred the chicken meat and discard the bones.

6. Return the shredded chicken to the pot. Add frozen peas and heavy cream (if using). Stir to combine and simmer for an additional 10 minutes.

7. Taste the chicken stew and adjust the seasoning if needed. Garnish with fresh parsley.

For the Dumplings:

1. In a mixing bowl, whisk together flour, baking powder, and salt.

2. Gradually add milk and melted butter to the dry ingredients, stirring until just combined. The dough will be sticky.

3. Drop spoonfuls of the dumpling dough onto the simmering chicken stew. Cover the pot and let the dumplings steam for 15-20 minutes until they are cooked through.

4. Serve the chicken and dumplings hot, with the dumplings nestled in the flavorful stew.

5. Enjoy this classic and comforting chicken and dumplings dish!

Irish Lamb Stew:

Ingredients:

- 2 pounds lamb stew meat, cut into cubes
- 2 tablespoons vegetable oil
- Salt and black pepper to taste
- 1/3 cup all-purpose flour
- 2 onions, chopped
- 3 carrots, sliced

- 3 celery stalks, sliced
- 3 cloves garlic, minced
- 4 cups beef or lamb broth
- 2 bay leaves
- 1 teaspoon dried thyme
- 1 teaspoon dried rosemary
- 1 1/2 pounds potatoes, peeled and diced
- Fresh parsley for garnish

Instructions:

1. In a large pot, heat vegetable oil over medium-high heat. Season lamb stew meat with salt and black pepper, then coat with flour.
2. Brown the lamb cubes in the pot on all sides. Work in batches to avoid overcrowding the pot. Remove the browned lamb and set it aside.
3. In the same pot, add chopped onions, sliced carrots, and sliced celery. Sauté for 5-7 minutes until the vegetables are softened.
4. Add minced garlic to the pot and cook for an additional 1-2 minutes until fragrant.
5. Return the browned lamb to the pot. Pour in beef or lamb broth, add bay leaves, dried thyme, and dried rosemary. Bring the mixture to a simmer.
6. Cover the pot and let the Irish lamb stew simmer for 1.5 to 2 hours, or until the lamb is tender.
7. Add diced potatoes to the pot and continue simmering for an additional 30-40 minutes until the potatoes are cooked through.
8. Taste the stew and adjust the seasoning if needed. Remove bay leaves.
9. Ladle the Irish lamb stew into bowls, garnish with fresh parsley, and serve hot.
10. Enjoy this hearty and flavorful Irish lamb stew as a comforting and satisfying meal.

Vegetarian Goulash:

Ingredients:

- 2 tablespoons vegetable oil
- 1 large onion, chopped
- 2 cloves garlic, minced
- 2 red bell peppers, diced
- 2 carrots, sliced
- 2 potatoes, peeled and diced
- 2 tablespoons tomato paste
- 1 can (14 oz) diced tomatoes
- 2 teaspoons paprika
- 1 teaspoon caraway seeds
- 1 teaspoon dried thyme
- 2 bay leaves
- Salt and black pepper to taste
- 3 cups vegetable broth
- 1 can (14 oz) kidney beans, drained and rinsed
- 1 cup frozen peas
- Fresh parsley for garnish
- Sour cream or yogurt for serving (optional)

Instructions:

1. In a large pot, heat vegetable oil over medium heat. Add chopped onion and sauté for 5-7 minutes until softened.
2. Add minced garlic to the pot and cook for an additional 1-2 minutes until fragrant.
3. Stir in diced red bell peppers, sliced carrots, and diced potatoes. Cook for 5-7 minutes, allowing the vegetables to slightly soften.
4. Add tomato paste to the pot and cook for 2-3 minutes to enhance its flavor.
5. Pour in diced tomatoes with their juice, paprika, caraway seeds, dried thyme, bay leaves, salt, and black pepper. Mix well.
6. Add vegetable broth to the pot and bring the mixture to a simmer.

7. Cover the pot and let the vegetarian goulash simmer for 20-25 minutes until the vegetables are tender.

8. Stir in kidney beans and frozen peas. Cook for an additional 5 minutes until the peas are heated through.

9. Taste the goulash and adjust the seasoning if needed. Remove bay leaves.

10. Ladle the vegetarian goulash into bowls, garnish with fresh parsley, and serve hot.

11. Optionally, serve with a dollop of sour cream or yogurt on top.

Seafood Stew:

Ingredients:

- 1 pound mixed seafood (shrimp, mussels, squid, fish fillets, etc.)
- 2 tablespoons olive oil
- 1 onion, chopped
- 3 cloves garlic, minced
- 1 bell pepper, diced
- 1 carrot, sliced
- 1 celery stalk, sliced
- 1 can (14 oz) diced tomatoes
- 1 cup fish or seafood broth
- 1/2 cup white wine (optional)
- 1 teaspoon dried thyme
- 1 teaspoon dried oregano
- 1 bay leaf
- Salt and black pepper to taste
- Pinch of red pepper flakes (optional, for heat)
- 1/2 cup chopped fresh parsley
- Crusty bread for serving

Instructions:

1. Clean and prepare the seafood. If using mussels, scrub the shells and debeard them. If using squid, clean and slice into rings. Pat dry fish fillets and shrimp.
2. In a large pot, heat olive oil over medium heat. Add chopped onion, minced garlic, diced bell pepper, sliced carrot, and sliced celery. Sauté for 5-7 minutes until the vegetables are softened.
3. Pour in diced tomatoes with their juice, fish or seafood broth, and white wine (if using). Add dried thyme, dried oregano, bay leaf, salt, black pepper, and red pepper flakes (if using). Mix well.
4. Bring the mixture to a simmer and let it cook for 10-15 minutes, allowing the flavors to meld.
5. Add the mixed seafood to the pot. Cook for 5-7 minutes until the seafood is cooked through. Be careful not to overcook.
6. Taste the seafood stew and adjust the seasoning if needed. Remove the bay leaf.
7. Stir in chopped fresh parsley.
8. Ladle the seafood stew into bowls and serve hot, accompanied by crusty bread.

Moroccan Chickpea Stew:

Ingredients:

- 2 tablespoons olive oil
- 1 onion, finely chopped
- 3 cloves garlic, minced
- 1 teaspoon ground cumin
- 1 teaspoon ground coriander
- 1 teaspoon ground turmeric
- 1/2 teaspoon ground cinnamon
- 1/4 teaspoon cayenne pepper (adjust to taste)
- 1 can (14 oz) diced tomatoes
- 1 can (14 oz) chickpeas, drained and rinsed
- 1 sweet potato, peeled and diced

- 1 carrot, sliced
- 1 zucchini, diced
- 4 cups vegetable broth
- Salt and black pepper to taste
- 1 cup couscous (optional, for serving)
- Fresh cilantro or parsley for garnish
- Lemon wedges for serving

Instructions:

1. In a large pot, heat olive oil over medium heat. Add chopped onion and sauté for 5-7 minutes until softened.
2. Add minced garlic to the pot and cook for an additional 1-2 minutes until fragrant.
3. Stir in ground cumin, ground coriander, ground turmeric, ground cinnamon, and cayenne pepper. Cook for 1-2 minutes to toast the spices.
4. Pour in diced tomatoes with their juice, drained chickpeas, diced sweet potato, sliced carrot, and diced zucchini. Mix well.
5. Add vegetable broth to the pot and bring the mixture to a simmer.
6. Cover the pot and let the Moroccan chickpea stew simmer for 20-25 minutes or until the vegetables are tender.
7. Season the stew with salt and black pepper to taste.
8. If using, prepare couscous according to package instructions.
9. Serve the Moroccan chickpea stew over couscous, if desired.
10. Garnish with fresh cilantro or parsley.
11. Serve hot with lemon wedges on the side.

Pork and Sweet Potato Stew:

Ingredients:

- 1.5 pounds pork shoulder, cut into cubes
- 2 tablespoons vegetable oil
- 1 onion, chopped

- 3 cloves garlic, minced
- 1 teaspoon smoked paprika
- 1 teaspoon ground cumin
- 1 teaspoon dried thyme
- Salt and black pepper to taste
- 2 tablespoons tomato paste
- 1 cup chicken broth
- 1 can (14 oz) diced tomatoes
- 2 sweet potatoes, peeled and diced
- 2 carrots, sliced
- 2 cups chicken broth
- 1 bay leaf
- Fresh parsley for garnish

Instructions:

1. In a large pot, heat vegetable oil over medium-high heat. Add cubed pork and brown on all sides. Remove the pork from the pot and set it aside.
2. In the same pot, add chopped onion and sauté for 5-7 minutes until softened.
3. Add minced garlic to the pot and cook for an additional 1-2 minutes until fragrant.
4. Stir in smoked paprika, ground cumin, dried thyme, salt, and black pepper. Cook for 1-2 minutes to toast the spices.
5. Add tomato paste to the pot and cook for an additional 2-3 minutes to enhance its flavor.
6. Pour in chicken broth, diced tomatoes with their juice, diced sweet potatoes, sliced carrots, and browned pork. Mix well.
7. Add additional chicken broth to the pot, ensuring that the ingredients are covered with liquid. Add a bay leaf.
8. Bring the stew to a simmer, cover the pot, and let it cook for 1.5 to 2 hours, or until the pork is tender and the flavors meld.
9. Taste the stew and adjust the seasoning if needed. Remove the bay leaf.

10. Ladle the pork and sweet potato stew into bowls, garnish with fresh parsley, and serve hot.

11. Enjoy this hearty and flavorful pork and sweet potato stew as a comforting and satisfying meal.

Italian Sausage and Bean Stew:

Ingredients:

- 1 pound Italian sausage links, sliced
- 2 tablespoons olive oil
- 1 onion, chopped
- 3 cloves garlic, minced
- 1 bell pepper, diced
- 2 carrots, sliced
- 2 celery stalks, sliced
- 1 can (14 oz) diced tomatoes
- 2 cans (14 oz each) cannellini beans, drained and rinsed
- 4 cups chicken or vegetable broth
- 1 teaspoon dried oregano
- 1 teaspoon dried basil
- 1/2 teaspoon dried thyme
- Salt and black pepper to taste
- 1 bunch fresh spinach, chopped
- Grated Parmesan cheese for serving
- Fresh basil for garnish

Instructions:

1. In a large pot, heat olive oil over medium-high heat. Add sliced Italian sausage and brown on all sides. Remove the sausage from the pot and set it aside.

2. In the same pot, add chopped onion, minced garlic, diced bell pepper, sliced carrots, and sliced celery. Sauté for 5-7 minutes until the vegetables are softened.

3. Pour in diced tomatoes with their juice, drained cannellini beans, chicken or vegetable broth, dried oregano, dried basil, dried thyme, salt, and black pepper. Mix well.

4. Return the browned Italian sausage to the pot. Bring the mixture to a simmer.

5. Cover the pot and let the Italian sausage and bean stew simmer for 20-25 minutes, allowing the flavors to meld.

6. Stir in chopped fresh spinach and cook for an additional 3-5 minutes until the spinach is wilted.

7. Taste the stew and adjust the seasoning if needed.

8. Ladle the Italian sausage and bean stew into bowls, garnish with grated Parmesan cheese and fresh basil, and serve hot.

Vegetable Curry Stew:

Ingredients:

- 2 tablespoons vegetable oil
- 1 large onion, finely chopped
- 3 cloves garlic, minced
- 1 tablespoon ginger, grated
- 2 tablespoons curry powder
- 1 teaspoon ground cumin
- 1 teaspoon ground coriander
- 1/2 teaspoon turmeric
- 1/4 teaspoon cayenne pepper (adjust to taste)
- 4 cups mixed vegetables (e.g., carrots, potatoes, bell peppers, peas)
- 1 can (14 oz) diced tomatoes
- 1 can (14 oz) coconut milk
- 2 cups vegetable broth
- Salt and pepper to taste
- Fresh cilantro for garnish

Instructions:

1. In a large pot, heat the vegetable oil over medium heat. Add chopped onions and sauté until translucent.

2. Add minced garlic and grated ginger to the pot, sauté for an additional 1-2 minutes until fragrant.

3. Stir in curry powder, ground cumin, ground coriander, turmeric, and cayenne pepper. Cook for 1-2 minutes to toast the spices.

4. Add mixed vegetables to the pot and coat them with the spice mixture.

5. Pour in diced tomatoes, coconut milk, and vegetable broth. Bring the stew to a simmer.

6. Reduce heat to low, cover the pot, and let it simmer for 20-25 minutes or until the vegetables are tender.

7. Season with salt and pepper to taste. Adjust the spice level if needed.

8. Serve the vegetable curry stew over rice or with naan bread. Garnish with fresh cilantro.

Hungarian Goulash:

Ingredients:

- 2 tablespoons vegetable oil
- 2 pounds beef stew meat, cubed
- 2 large onions, finely chopped
- 3 cloves garlic, minced
- 2 tablespoons sweet paprika
- 1 teaspoon caraway seeds
- 1 teaspoon dried thyme
- 2 bay leaves
- 2 tablespoons tomato paste
- 2 large tomatoes, diced
- 3 cups beef broth

- Salt and pepper to taste
- 4 large potatoes, peeled and diced
- Chopped fresh parsley for garnish

Instructions:

1. In a large pot or Dutch oven, heat vegetable oil over medium-high heat. Add cubed beef and brown on all sides. Remove beef and set aside.

2. In the same pot, add chopped onions and sauté until softened. Add minced garlic and sauté for an additional minute.

3. Stir in sweet paprika, caraway seeds, dried thyme, and bay leaves. Cook for 1-2 minutes to release the flavors.

4. Add tomato paste and diced tomatoes to the pot. Cook for another 2-3 minutes.

5. Return the browned beef to the pot. Pour in beef broth, season with salt and pepper, and bring the mixture to a boil.

6. Reduce the heat to low, cover, and simmer for 1.5 to 2 hours or until the beef is tender.

7. Add diced potatoes to the pot and continue to simmer until the potatoes are cooked through.

8. Adjust salt and pepper if needed. Remove bay leaves.

9. Serve the Hungarian Goulash hot, garnished with chopped fresh parsley.

White Bean and Kale Stew:

Ingredients:

- 2 tablespoons olive oil
- 1 onion, diced
- 2 carrots, sliced
- 3 cloves garlic, minced
- 1 teaspoon dried thyme
- 1 teaspoon dried rosemary
- 2 cans (15 oz each) white beans, drained and rinsed

- 4 cups vegetable broth
- 1 can (14 oz) diced tomatoes
- 1 bunch kale, stems removed and leaves chopped
- Salt and pepper to taste
- Parmesan cheese (optional, for serving)

Instructions:

1. In a large pot, heat olive oil over medium heat. Add diced onion and sliced carrots, sauté until softened.
2. Add minced garlic, dried thyme, and dried rosemary. Sauté for an additional 1-2 minutes until fragrant.
3. Pour in white beans, vegetable broth, and diced tomatoes with their juice. Bring the mixture to a simmer.
4. Reduce heat to low, add chopped kale to the pot. Simmer for about 15-20 minutes until the kale is tender.
5. Season the stew with salt and pepper to taste. Adjust as needed.
6. Optional: Serve the stew hot, garnished with Parmesan cheese if desired.

Spanish Chicken and Chorizo Stew:

Ingredients:

- 2 tablespoons olive oil
- 4 bone-in, skin-on chicken thighs
- Salt and pepper to taste
- 1 onion, finely chopped
- 1 red bell pepper, diced
- 1 yellow bell pepper, diced
- 3 cloves garlic, minced
- 1 teaspoon smoked paprika
- 1 teaspoon ground cumin
- 1 teaspoon dried oregano

- 1/2 teaspoon cayenne pepper (adjust to taste)
- 1 cup chorizo sausage, sliced
- 1 can (14 oz) diced tomatoes
- 1 cup chicken broth
- 1/2 cup dry white wine (optional)
- 1 cup frozen peas
- Fresh parsley, chopped (for garnish)

Instructions:

1. In a large, oven-safe pot, heat olive oil over medium-high heat. Season chicken thighs with salt and pepper, then brown them on both sides. Remove and set aside.
2. In the same pot, add chopped onion and diced bell peppers. Sauté until softened.
3. Add minced garlic, smoked paprika, ground cumin, dried oregano, and cayenne pepper. Stir well and cook for 1-2 minutes.
4. Add sliced chorizo to the pot and cook for an additional 2-3 minutes.
5. Pour in diced tomatoes with their juice, chicken broth, and white wine (if using). Bring the mixture to a simmer.
6. Return the browned chicken thighs to the pot, ensuring they are partially submerged in the liquid. Cover the pot and transfer it to a preheated oven at 350°F (180°C). Bake for 30-40 minutes or until the chicken is cooked through.
7. Remove the pot from the oven and stir in frozen peas. Let it sit for a couple of minutes until the peas are heated through.
8. Garnish with chopped fresh parsley before serving.

Black Bean and Quinoa Stew:

Ingredients:

- 1 cup quinoa, rinsed
- 2 tablespoons olive oil
- 1 onion, finely chopped
- 2 bell peppers (any color), diced

- 3 cloves garlic, minced
- 1 teaspoon ground cumin
- 1 teaspoon chili powder
- 1 teaspoon smoked paprika
- 2 cans (15 oz each) black beans, drained and rinsed
- 1 can (14 oz) diced tomatoes
- 4 cups vegetable broth
- 1 cup frozen corn
- Salt and pepper to taste
- Juice of 1 lime
- Fresh cilantro, chopped (for garnish)
- Avocado slices (optional, for serving)

Instructions:

1. Cook quinoa according to package instructions. Set aside.
2. In a large pot, heat olive oil over medium heat. Add chopped onion and diced bell peppers. Sauté until softened.
3. Add minced garlic, ground cumin, chili powder, and smoked paprika. Cook for an additional 1-2 minutes until fragrant.
4. Stir in black beans, diced tomatoes, and vegetable broth. Bring the stew to a simmer.
5. Add frozen corn to the pot. Season with salt and pepper to taste.
6. Simmer the stew for about 15-20 minutes to allow the flavors to meld.
7. Stir in cooked quinoa and lime juice. Adjust seasoning if needed.
8. Serve the Black Bean and Quinoa Stew hot, garnished with chopped fresh cilantro. Optionally, top with avocado slices.

Venison Stew:

Ingredients:

- 2 pounds venison stew meat, cubed

- 2 tablespoons vegetable oil
- Salt and pepper to taste
- 1 onion, finely chopped
- 3 cloves garlic, minced
- 2 carrots, sliced
- 2 celery stalks, chopped
- 1 cup red wine (optional)
- 4 cups beef or venison broth
- 2 bay leaves
- 1 teaspoon dried thyme
- 1 teaspoon rosemary, chopped
- 1 pound potatoes, peeled and diced
- 1 cup mushrooms, sliced
- 1 cup frozen peas
- Fresh parsley, chopped (for garnish)

Instructions:

1. In a large pot, heat vegetable oil over medium-high heat. Season venison cubes with salt and pepper, then brown them on all sides. Remove and set aside.
2. In the same pot, add chopped onion, minced garlic, sliced carrots, and chopped celery. Sauté until vegetables are softened.
3. Pour in red wine (if using), scraping the bottom of the pot to release any browned bits.
4. Return the browned venison to the pot. Add beef or venison broth, bay leaves, dried thyme, and chopped rosemary. Bring the stew to a simmer.
5. Reduce heat to low, cover the pot, and let it simmer for 1.5 to 2 hours or until the venison is tender.
6. Add diced potatoes, sliced mushrooms, and frozen peas to the pot. Continue simmering until the vegetables are cooked through.
7. Adjust salt and pepper to taste. Remove bay leaves.

8. Serve the Venison Stew hot, garnished with chopped fresh parsley.

Turkish Eggplant and Chickpea Stew:

Ingredients:

- 2 large eggplants, diced
- Salt for sweating the eggplants
- 3 tablespoons olive oil
- 1 onion, finely chopped
- 3 cloves garlic, minced
- 1 red bell pepper, diced
- 1 green bell pepper, diced
- 1 can (15 oz) chickpeas, drained and rinsed
- 2 large tomatoes, diced
- 2 tablespoons tomato paste
- 1 teaspoon ground cumin
- 1 teaspoon paprika
- 1/2 teaspoon red pepper flakes (adjust to taste)
- 1 cup vegetable broth
- Salt and pepper to taste
- Fresh parsley, chopped (for garnish)
- Yogurt (optional, for serving)

Instructions:

1. Dice the eggplants, sprinkle with salt, and let them sit for about 30 minutes to draw out excess moisture. Rinse and pat dry.
2. In a large pot, heat olive oil over medium heat. Add chopped onion and sauté until softened.
3. Add minced garlic, diced red and green bell peppers, and diced eggplants to the pot. Sauté until the vegetables are tender.
4. Stir in chickpeas, diced tomatoes, and tomato paste. Cook for 2-3 minutes.

5. Add ground cumin, paprika, and red pepper flakes. Mix well to coat the vegetables and chickpeas with the spices.

6. Pour in vegetable broth, season with salt and pepper, and bring the stew to a simmer.

7. Cover the pot and let it simmer for 20-25 minutes or until the flavors meld and the vegetables are cooked.

8. Adjust salt and pepper to taste. Serve the Turkish Eggplant and Chickpea Stew hot, garnished with chopped fresh parsley. Optionally, serve with a dollop of yogurt on top.

CHAPTER 10: WEEKLY MEAL PLAN AND PREPARATION

Day 1:

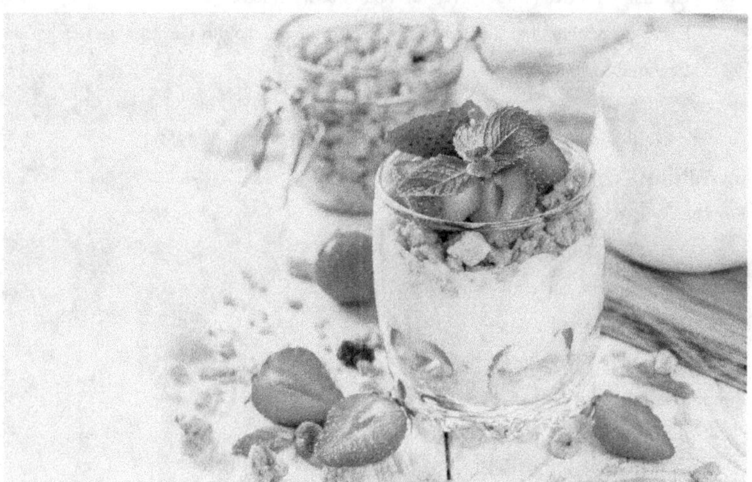

Breakfast: Greek Yogurt Parfait with Berries and Granola

Ingredients:

- 1 cup Greek yogurt
- 1 cup mixed berries (strawberries, blueberries, raspberries)
- 1/2 cup granola
- 1 tablespoon honey (optional)
- Fresh mint leaves for garnish (optional)

Instructions:

1. In a glass or a bowl, layer 1/4 cup of Greek yogurt at the bottom.
2. Add a layer of mixed berries on top of the yogurt.
3. Sprinkle 2 tablespoons of granola over the berries.

4. Repeat the layers until the glass or bowl is filled, finishing with a final layer of berries and granola on top.

5. Drizzle honey over the top for added sweetness if desired.

6. Garnish with fresh mint leaves for a burst of freshness.

7. Serve immediately and enjoy your delicious Greek Yogurt Parfait with Berries and Granola!

Lunch: Grilled Chicken Salad with Mixed Greens and Veggies

Ingredients:

For the Grilled Chicken:

- 2 boneless, skinless chicken breasts
- 2 tablespoons olive oil
- 1 teaspoon dried oregano
- Salt and pepper to taste

For the Salad:

- 6 cups mixed salad greens (e.g., spinach, arugula, romaine)
- 1 cucumber, sliced
- 1 cup cherry tomatoes, halved
- 1 bell pepper, thinly sliced
- 1/2 red onion, thinly sliced
- 1/4 cup Kalamata olives, pitted and sliced
- 1/2 cup feta cheese, crumbled

For the Dressing:

- 3 tablespoons extra-virgin olive oil
- 2 tablespoons red wine vinegar
- 1 teaspoon Dijon mustard
- 1 clove garlic, minced
- Salt and pepper to taste

Instructions:

1. Preheat the grill to medium-high heat.

2. In a bowl, combine olive oil, dried oregano, salt, and pepper. Coat the chicken breasts with this mixture.

3. Grill the chicken for about 6-8 minutes per side or until cooked through. Let it rest for a few minutes before slicing.

4. In a large salad bowl, combine the mixed greens, cucumber, cherry tomatoes, bell pepper, red onion, Kalamata olives, and feta cheese.

5. In a small bowl, whisk together the dressing ingredients: olive oil, red wine vinegar, Dijon mustard, minced garlic, salt, and pepper.

6. Slice the grilled chicken and arrange it on top of the salad.

7. Drizzle the dressing over the salad and chicken.

8. Toss the salad gently to coat everything with the dressing.

9. Serve the Grilled Chicken Salad immediately, and enjoy a flavorful and healthy lunch!

Snack: Sliced Apple with Almond Butter

Ingredients:

- 1 apple, cored and sliced
- 2 tablespoons almond butter

Instructions:

1. Wash and core the apple, then slice it into thin wedges.

2. In a small bowl, scoop out 2 tablespoons of almond butter.

3. Dip each apple slice into the almond butter or spread almond butter on each slice.

4. Arrange the apple slices on a plate.

5. Optional: Sprinkle a pinch of cinnamon or drizzle honey on top for added flavor.

6. Enjoy your simple and healthy snack of Sliced Apple with Almond Butter!

Dinner: Baked Lemon Herb Salmon with Quinoa and Roasted Vegetables

Ingredients:

For the Salmon:

- 4 salmon fillets
- 2 tablespoons olive oil
- 2 tablespoons fresh lemon juice
- 1 teaspoon dried thyme
- 1 teaspoon dried rosemary
- Salt and pepper to taste
- Lemon slices for garnish

For the Quinoa:

- 1 cup quinoa, rinsed
- 2 cups vegetable broth or water
- Salt to taste

For the Roasted Vegetables:

- 1 zucchini, sliced
- 1 bell pepper (any color), sliced
- 1 cup cherry tomatoes
- 1 red onion, sliced
- 2 tablespoons olive oil
- 1 teaspoon dried oregano
- Salt and pepper to taste

Instructions:

1. Preheat the oven: Preheat the oven to 400°F (200°C).
2. Prepare the Salmon:
   - In a small bowl, mix olive oil, lemon juice, dried thyme, dried rosemary, salt, and pepper.
   - Place the salmon fillets on a baking sheet lined with parchment paper.
   - Brush the salmon fillets with the lemon herb mixture.
   - Place lemon slices on top of each fillet.

- ○ Bake in the preheated oven for 15-20 minutes or until the salmon is cooked through.

3. Prepare the Quinoa:
   - ○ In a saucepan, combine quinoa and vegetable broth (or water).
   - ○ Bring to a boil, then reduce heat to low, cover, and simmer for 15 minutes or until the quinoa is cooked and water is absorbed.
   - ○ Fluff the quinoa with a fork and season with salt to taste.

4. Prepare the Roasted Vegetables:
   - ○ In a bowl, toss zucchini, bell pepper, cherry tomatoes, and red onion with olive oil, dried oregano, salt, and pepper.
   - ○ Spread the vegetables on a baking sheet and roast in the oven for 20-25 minutes or until they are tender and slightly caramelized.

5. Assemble the Dinner:
   - ○ Serve the baked lemon herb salmon over a bed of quinoa.
   - ○ Arrange the roasted vegetables on the side.
   - ○ Garnish with additional lemon slices.
   - ○ Enjoy your wholesome and flavorful dinner!

Day 2:

Breakfast: Oatmeal with Sliced Banana and Almond Butter

Ingredients:

- 1/2 cup old-fashioned rolled oats
- 1 cup milk (dairy or plant-based)
- Pinch of salt
- 1 banana, sliced
- 1 tablespoon almond butter
- Optional toppings: honey, chia seeds, chopped nuts

Instructions:

1. Cook the Oatmeal:
    o In a saucepan, combine the rolled oats, milk, and a pinch of salt.
    o Bring the mixture to a gentle boil over medium heat, stirring occasionally.
    o Reduce the heat to low and simmer for 5-7 minutes or until the oatmeal reaches your desired consistency.
2. Prepare the Toppings:
    o While the oatmeal is cooking, slice the banana.
3. Assemble the Breakfast:
    o Once the oatmeal is ready, pour it into a bowl.
    o Top with sliced bananas and a dollop of almond butter.
4. Optional: Add More Toppings:
    o Drizzle with honey for added sweetness.
    o Sprinkle with chia seeds or chopped nuts for extra texture and nutrients.
5. Enjoy your Oatmeal with Sliced Banana and Almond Butter!

Lunch: Quinoa and Black Bean Bowl with Avocado

Ingredients:

For the Quinoa and Black Bean Base:

- 1 cup quinoa, rinsed
- 2 cups vegetable broth or water
- 1 can (15 oz) black beans, drained and rinsed
- 1 teaspoon ground cumin
- 1 teaspoon chili powder
- Salt and pepper to taste

For the Avocado Topping:

- 1 ripe avocado, sliced
- Juice of 1 lime
- Salt to taste

Optional Bowl Additions:

- Cherry tomatoes, halved
- Corn kernels (fresh, canned, or frozen)
- Red onion, finely diced
- Fresh cilantro, chopped
- Hot sauce or salsa

Instructions:

1. Cook the Quinoa and Black Bean Base:
   - In a saucepan, combine quinoa and vegetable broth (or water).
   - Bring to a boil, then reduce heat to low, cover, and simmer for 15 minutes or until quinoa is cooked and liquid is absorbed.
   - In a separate pan, heat black beans with ground cumin, chili powder, salt, and pepper.
2. Prepare the Avocado Topping:
   - In a bowl, gently toss avocado slices with lime juice and a pinch of salt.
3. Assemble the Quinoa and Black Bean Bowl:
   - Divide the cooked quinoa and black beans among serving bowls.
4. Add Bowl Toppings:
   - Arrange avocado slices on top of each bowl.
   - Add cherry tomatoes, corn kernels, diced red onion, and chopped cilantro.
5. Optional: Add Hot Sauce or Salsa:
   - Drizzle with hot sauce or salsa for an extra kick.

Snack: Hummus with Veggie Sticks

Ingredients:

- 1 cup hummus (store-bought or homemade)
- Carrot sticks
- Celery sticks
- Cucumber slices
- Bell pepper strips (any color)

- Cherry tomatoes, halved

Instructions:

1. Prepare the Hummus:
   - If using store-bought hummus, transfer it to a serving bowl. If making homemade hummus, follow your preferred recipe and prepare it in advance.
2. Wash and Cut the Veggies:
   - Wash and cut carrot sticks, celery sticks, cucumber slices, bell pepper strips, and halve cherry tomatoes.
3. Arrange and Serve:
   - Arrange the veggie sticks around the bowl of hummus on a serving platter.

Dinner: Turkey and Vegetable Skewers with Brown Rice

Ingredients:

For the Turkey Skewers:

- 1 pound turkey breast or turkey tenderloin, cut into cubes
- 2 tablespoons olive oil
- 1 tablespoon lemon juice
- 2 cloves garlic, minced
- 1 teaspoon dried oregano
- 1 teaspoon smoked paprika
- Salt and pepper to taste

For the Vegetable Skewers:

- Cherry tomatoes
- Bell peppers (any color), cut into chunks
- Red onion, cut into wedges

For the Brown Rice:

- 1 cup brown rice
- 2 cups water or chicken broth
- Salt to taste

For the Yogurt Sauce:

- 1/2 cup Greek yogurt
- 1 tablespoon fresh lemon juice
- 1 tablespoon fresh dill, chopped
- Salt and pepper to taste

Instructions:

1. Marinate the Turkey:
   - In a bowl, mix olive oil, lemon juice, minced garlic, dried oregano, smoked paprika, salt, and pepper.
   - Add the turkey cubes to the marinade, ensuring they are well coated. Let it marinate for at least 30 minutes.
2. Preheat the Grill or Oven:
   - Preheat the grill or oven to medium-high heat.
3. Prepare the Skewers:
   - Thread the marinated turkey cubes onto skewers alternately with cherry tomatoes, bell peppers, and red onion wedges.
4. Grill or Bake:
   - Grill the skewers for about 10-15 minutes, turning occasionally until the turkey is cooked through and the vegetables are slightly charred.
   - Alternatively, you can bake the skewers in the oven at 400°F (200°C) for about 20-25 minutes.
5. Prepare the Brown Rice:
   - In a separate pot, combine brown rice, water or chicken broth, and a pinch of salt.
   - Bring to a boil, then reduce heat to low, cover, and simmer for 45-50 minutes or until the rice is cooked.
6. Make the Yogurt Sauce:
   - In a small bowl, mix Greek yogurt, fresh lemon juice, chopped fresh dill, salt, and pepper.

7. Serve:

- Serve the Turkey and Vegetable Skewers over a bed of brown rice.
- Drizzle with the yogurt sauce.

Day 3:

Breakfast: Smoothie Bowl with Spinach, Berries, and Chia Seeds

Ingredients:

For the Smoothie Base:

- 1 cup fresh spinach leaves
- 1/2 banana, frozen
- 1/2 cup mixed berries (strawberries, blueberries, raspberries)
- 1/2 cup Greek yogurt
- 1/2 cup almond milk (or any milk of your choice)
- 1 tablespoon chia seeds

Toppings:

- Sliced strawberries
- Blueberries
- Chia seeds
- Granola
- Shredded coconut

Instructions:

1. Prepare the Smoothie Base:
   - In a blender, combine fresh spinach, frozen banana, mixed berries, Greek yogurt, almond milk, and chia seeds.
   - Blend until smooth and creamy.
2. Assemble the Smoothie Bowl:
   - Pour the smoothie into a bowl.
3. Add Toppings:

- Top the smoothie bowl with sliced strawberries, blueberries, additional chia seeds, granola, and shredded coconut.

4. Customize:
   - Feel free to get creative with additional toppings like nuts, seeds, or drizzles of honey.

Lunch: Lentil Soup with a Side of Mixed Greens

Ingredients:

- 1 cup dried green or brown lentils, rinsed and drained
- 1 tablespoon olive oil
- 1 onion, finely chopped
- 2 carrots, diced
- 2 celery stalks, diced
- 3 cloves garlic, minced
- 1 teaspoon ground cumin
- 1 teaspoon ground coriander
- 1/2 teaspoon smoked paprika
- 1 can (14 oz) diced tomatoes
- 6 cups vegetable or chicken broth
- Salt and pepper to taste
- Fresh lemon juice (optional, for serving)
- Fresh parsley, chopped (for garnish)

Instructions:

1. Prepare Lentils:
   - Rinse lentils under cold water and set aside.
2. Sauté Vegetables:
   - In a large pot, heat olive oil over medium heat. Add chopped onion, diced carrots, and diced celery. Sauté until vegetables are softened.
3. Add Aromatics and Spices:

- Add minced garlic, ground cumin, ground coriander, and smoked paprika. Stir and cook for 1-2 minutes until fragrant.

4. Simmer the Soup:

   - Pour in diced tomatoes and broth. Add rinsed lentils. Bring the mixture to a boil, then reduce heat to low, cover, and simmer for about 20-25 minutes or until lentils are tender.

5. Season and Serve:

   - Season the soup with salt and pepper to taste. Add more broth if needed. If desired, squeeze fresh lemon juice into the soup for brightness.

6. Garnish:

   - Ladle the lentil soup into bowls. Garnish with chopped fresh parsley.

Mixed Greens:

Ingredients:

- Mixed salad greens (e.g., spinach, arugula, romaine)
- Cherry tomatoes, halved
- Cucumber, sliced
- Balsamic vinaigrette dressing

Instructions:

1. Assemble Salad:

   - In a bowl, combine mixed salad greens, halved cherry tomatoes, and sliced cucumber.

2. Dress the Salad:

   - Drizzle balsamic vinaigrette dressing over the salad and toss gently to coat.

3. Serve:

   - Serve the Lentil Soup with a side of Mixed Greens for a balanced and satisfying lunch.

Snack: Mixed Nuts

Ingredients:

- 1 cup raw almonds
- 1 cup raw walnuts
- 1/2 cup raw cashews
- 1/2 cup raw pecans
- 1/4 cup raw pumpkin seeds
- 1/4 cup raw sunflower seeds
- 1 tablespoon olive oil
- 1 teaspoon sea salt (adjust to taste)
- 1/2 teaspoon ground cumin (optional)
- 1/2 teaspoon paprika (optional)
- 1/4 teaspoon cayenne pepper (optional, for a spicy kick)

Instructions:

1. Preheat the Oven:
   - Preheat your oven to 350°F (175°C).
2. Mix the Nuts:
   - In a large bowl, combine almonds, walnuts, cashews, pecans, pumpkin seeds, and sunflower seeds.
3. Add Olive Oil and Seasonings:
   - Drizzle olive oil over the mixed nuts and toss to coat evenly.
   - If desired, add sea salt, ground cumin, paprika, and cayenne pepper. Toss again to evenly distribute the seasonings.
4. Spread on Baking Sheet:
   - Spread the seasoned nuts in a single layer on a baking sheet lined with parchment paper.
5. Roast in the Oven:
   - Roast the nuts in the preheated oven for 10-15 minutes or until they are golden and fragrant, stirring once or twice during the baking time.
6. Cool and Store:

- Allow the mixed nuts to cool completely before transferring them to an airtight container.

Dinner: Eggplant Parmesan with a Side Salad

Ingredients:

- 2 large eggplants, sliced into 1/2-inch rounds
- Salt, for sweating the eggplant
- 2 cups breadcrumbs (seasoned or plain)
- 1 cup grated Parmesan cheese
- 3 large eggs, beaten
- 2 cups marinara sauce
- 2 cups shredded mozzarella cheese
- Fresh basil leaves, for garnish (optional)

Instructions:

1. Preheat the Oven:
   - Preheat your oven to 375°F (190°C).
2. Prepare the Eggplant:
   - Sprinkle salt on the eggplant slices and let them sit for 30 minutes to release excess moisture. Pat them dry with a paper towel.
3. Bread and Bake:
   - In one bowl, place breadcrumbs. In another bowl, mix grated Parmesan cheese. Dip each eggplant slice first in the beaten eggs, then in the breadcrumbs and Parmesan mixture, coating evenly.
   - Place the breaded eggplant slices on a baking sheet lined with parchment paper.
   - Bake for about 20-25 minutes or until the eggplant is golden brown and cooked through.
4. Assemble Eggplant Parmesan:
   - In a baking dish, spread a thin layer of marinara sauce.

- ○ Arrange a layer of baked eggplant slices on top of the sauce.
- ○ Sprinkle with mozzarella cheese and repeat the layers until all ingredients are used, finishing with a layer of cheese on top.

5. Bake Until Bubbly:
- ○ Bake in the preheated oven for 25-30 minutes or until the cheese is melted, bubbly, and golden.

6. Garnish and Serve:
- ○ Garnish with fresh basil leaves if desired.
- ○ Allow the Eggplant Parmesan to cool slightly before serving.

Side Salad:

Ingredients:

- Mixed salad greens (e.g., arugula, spinach, romaine)
- Cherry tomatoes, halved
- Cucumber, sliced
- Red onion, thinly sliced
- Balsamic vinaigrette dressing

Instructions:

1. Assemble Salad:
- ○ In a bowl, combine mixed salad greens, cherry tomatoes, cucumber, and thinly sliced red onion.

2. Dress the Salad:
- ○ Drizzle balsamic vinaigrette dressing over the salad and toss gently to coat.

3. Serve:
- ○ Serve the Eggplant Parmesan with a side of the refreshing Mixed Salad for a delightful and satisfying dinner.

Day 4:

Breakfast: Whole Grain Toast with Mashed Avocado

Ingredients:

- 2 slices whole grain bread
- 1 ripe avocado
- Salt and pepper to taste
- Red pepper flakes (optional, for a bit of heat)
- Lemon juice (optional, for added freshness)
- Optional toppings: poached egg, cherry tomatoes, feta cheese, or radish slices

Instructions:

1. Toast the Bread:
   - Toast the slices of whole grain bread to your desired level of crispiness.
2. Prepare the Avocado:
   - Cut the ripe avocado in half and remove the pit. Scoop the flesh into a bowl.
3. Mash the Avocado:
   - Mash the avocado using a fork until it reaches your preferred level of creaminess.
4. Season the Avocado:
   - Add salt and pepper to taste. For extra flavor, you can also sprinkle red pepper flakes and a splash of lemon juice.
5. Spread on Toast:
   - Spread the mashed avocado evenly over the toasted whole grain bread slices.
6. Optional Toppings:
   - Customize your avocado toast with additional toppings like a poached egg, sliced cherry tomatoes, crumbled feta cheese, or radish slices.

Lunch: Chickpea Salad with Cucumber and Feta

Ingredients:

For the Salad:

- 1 can (15 oz) chickpeas, drained and rinsed
- 1 cucumber, diced
- 1/2 red onion, finely chopped
- 1 cup cherry tomatoes, halved
- 1/2 cup crumbled feta cheese
- 1/4 cup Kalamata olives, pitted and sliced
- Fresh parsley, chopped (for garnish)

For the Dressing:

- 3 tablespoons extra-virgin olive oil
- 2 tablespoons red wine vinegar
- 1 teaspoon Dijon mustard
- 1 clove garlic, minced
- Salt and pepper to taste

Instructions:

1. Prepare Chickpeas:
   - Drain and rinse chickpeas under cold water.
2. Assemble Salad:
   - In a large bowl, combine chickpeas, diced cucumber, chopped red onion, cherry tomatoes, crumbled feta cheese, and sliced Kalamata olives.
3. Make the Dressing:
   - In a small bowl, whisk together olive oil, red wine vinegar, Dijon mustard, minced garlic, salt, and pepper.
4. Dress the Salad:
   - Pour the dressing over the salad and toss gently to coat all the ingredients.
5. Garnish:
   - Garnish the Chickpea Salad with chopped fresh parsley.

6. Chill and Serve:

   o   Refrigerate the salad for at least 30 minutes before serving to allow the
       flavors to meld.

Snack: Cottage Cheese with Pineapple

Ingredients:

- 1 cup cottage cheese
- 1 cup fresh pineapple chunks (or canned pineapple tidbits, drained)
- Honey or agave syrup (optional, for drizzling)
- Mint leaves for garnish (optional)

Instructions:

1. Prepare Cottage Cheese:

   o   Scoop 1 cup of cottage cheese into a bowl.

2. Add Pineapple Chunks:

   o   Add 1 cup of fresh pineapple chunks to the cottage cheese.

3. Optional Sweetener:

   o   If you desire added sweetness, drizzle honey or agave syrup over the
       cottage cheese and pineapple.

4. Gently Mix:

   o   Gently mix the cottage cheese and pineapple to combine the flavors.

5. Garnish (Optional):

   o   Garnish with mint leaves for a fresh and aromatic touch.

Dinner: Shrimp and Zucchini Noodles in Olive Oil and Garlic

Ingredients:

- 1 pound large shrimp, peeled and deveined
- 4 medium zucchini, spiralized into noodles
- 3 tablespoons olive oil
- 4 cloves garlic, minced

- Red pepper flakes (optional, for heat)
- Salt and black pepper to taste
- 1 tablespoon lemon juice
- Fresh parsley, chopped (for garnish)

Instructions:

1. Prepare Shrimp:
   - Pat the shrimp dry and season with salt and black pepper.
2. Spiralize Zucchini:
   - Spiralize the zucchini into noodles using a spiralizer. Set aside.
3. Cook Shrimp:
   - In a large skillet, heat 2 tablespoons of olive oil over medium-high heat.
   - Add shrimp and cook for 2-3 minutes per side or until they turn pink and opaque. Remove shrimp from the skillet and set aside.
4. Cook Zucchini Noodles:
   - In the same skillet, add the remaining 1 tablespoon of olive oil.
   - Add minced garlic and red pepper flakes (if using). Sauté for about 1 minute until fragrant.
   - Add spiralized zucchini noodles and toss for 2-3 minutes until just tender. Be careful not to overcook, as zucchini noodles can become mushy quickly.
5. Combine Shrimp and Zucchini:
   - Return the cooked shrimp to the skillet with zucchini noodles.
   - Drizzle with lemon juice and toss everything together until well combined.
6. Adjust Seasonings:
   - Taste and adjust salt and pepper according to your preference.
7. Garnish and Serve:
   - Garnish with chopped fresh parsley.
   - Serve the Shrimp and Zucchini Noodles immediately while warm.

Breakfast: Scrambled Eggs with Spinach and Tomatoes

Ingredients:

- 4 large eggs
- 1 cup fresh spinach, chopped
- 1 cup cherry tomatoes, halved
- 1 tablespoon olive oil or butter
- Salt and black pepper to taste
- Optional toppings: feta cheese, avocado slices, hot sauce
- Fresh parsley or chives, chopped (for garnish)

Instructions:

1. Prepare Ingredients:
   - Whisk the eggs in a bowl and set aside.
   - Chop fresh spinach and halve cherry tomatoes.
2. Sauté Vegetables:
   - In a skillet, heat olive oil or butter over medium heat.
   - Add chopped spinach and cook for 1-2 minutes until wilted.
3. Add Tomatoes:
   - Add halved cherry tomatoes to the skillet and cook for an additional 1-2 minutes until slightly softened.
4. Scramble Eggs:
   - Push the vegetables to one side of the skillet and pour the whisked eggs into the empty side.
   - Allow the eggs to set for a moment, then gently scramble with a spatula.
5. Combine and Season:
   - Once the eggs are mostly set, combine them with the sautéed vegetables.
   - Season with salt and black pepper to taste.
6. Optional Toppings:

- ○ If desired, add toppings like feta cheese, avocado slices, or a drizzle of hot sauce.
7. Garnish and Serve:
   - ○ Garnish with chopped fresh parsley or chives.
   - ○ Serve the Scrambled Eggs with Spinach and Tomatoes warm.

Lunch: Quinoa Stuffed Bell Peppers with a Side of Greek Yogurt

Ingredients:

For the Quinoa Stuffed Bell Peppers:

- 4 large bell peppers, halved and seeds removed
- 1 cup quinoa, rinsed
- 2 cups vegetable broth or water
- 1 tablespoon olive oil
- 1 onion, finely chopped
- 2 cloves garlic, minced
- 1 zucchini, diced
- 1 cup cherry tomatoes, halved
- 1 cup black beans, drained and rinsed
- 1 teaspoon ground cumin
- 1 teaspoon smoked paprika
- Salt and pepper to taste
- 1 cup shredded cheese (cheddar, mozzarella, or your choice)

For the Side of Greek Yogurt:

- 1 cup Greek yogurt
- 1 tablespoon lemon juice
- 1 tablespoon fresh dill, chopped
- Salt and pepper to taste

Instructions:

1. Prepare Quinoa:

- In a saucepan, combine quinoa and vegetable broth (or water).
   - Bring to a boil, then reduce heat to low, cover, and simmer for 15 minutes or until quinoa is cooked and liquid is absorbed.
2. Preheat the Oven:
   - Preheat your oven to 375°F (190°C).
3. Sauté Vegetables:
   - In a large skillet, heat olive oil over medium heat.
   - Add chopped onion and garlic, sauté until softened.
   - Add diced zucchini, halved cherry tomatoes, black beans, ground cumin, smoked paprika, salt, and pepper. Cook for an additional 3-5 minutes until vegetables are tender.
4. Combine Quinoa and Vegetables:
   - Mix the cooked quinoa with the sautéed vegetables in the skillet.
5. Stuff Bell Peppers:
   - Place bell pepper halves on a baking dish.
   - Spoon the quinoa and vegetable mixture into each pepper half.
6. Add Cheese and Bake:
   - Sprinkle shredded cheese on top of each stuffed pepper.
   - Bake in the preheated oven for 20-25 minutes or until the cheese is melted and bubbly.
7. Prepare Greek Yogurt Side:
   - In a small bowl, mix Greek yogurt, lemon juice, chopped fresh dill, salt, and pepper.
8. Serve:
   - Serve the Quinoa Stuffed Bell Peppers with a dollop of the Greek yogurt mixture on the side.

Snack: Trail Mix with Nuts and Dried Fruits

Ingredients:

- 1 cup almonds
- 1 cup walnuts
- 1 cup cashews
- 1 cup dried cranberries
- 1/2 cup raisins
- 1/2 cup dried apricots, chopped
- 1/2 cup pumpkin seeds
- 1/2 cup dark chocolate chips (optional)
- 1/2 teaspoon sea salt (optional, for a sweet and salty mix)

Instructions:

1. Prepare Nuts:
   - If the nuts are raw, you can toast them for added flavor. Spread almonds, walnuts, and cashews on a baking sheet and roast in the oven at 350°F (175°C) for 8-10 minutes, or until they become fragrant. Allow them to cool.
2. Combine Ingredients:
   - In a large bowl, combine toasted nuts, dried cranberries, raisins, chopped dried apricots, pumpkin seeds, and dark chocolate chips (if using).
3. Optional Sweet and Salty Mix:
   - If you like a sweet and salty mix, sprinkle a small amount of sea salt over the mixture. Toss to combine.
4. Mix Thoroughly:
   - Mix all the ingredients thoroughly until well distributed.
5. Store:
   - Transfer the trail mix to an airtight container for storage.

Dinner: Grilled Vegetable and Chicken Kabobs with Quinoa

Ingredients:

For the Chicken Marinade:

- 1 pound boneless, skinless chicken breasts, cut into chunks
- 3 tablespoons olive oil
- 2 tablespoons soy sauce
- 2 cloves garlic, minced
- 1 teaspoon dried oregano
- 1 teaspoon paprika
- Salt and black pepper to taste

For the Kabobs:

- Bell peppers (assorted colors), cut into chunks
- Zucchini, sliced into rounds
- Red onion, cut into wedges
- Cherry tomatoes
- Wooden or metal skewers

For the Quinoa:

- 1 cup quinoa, rinsed
- 2 cups vegetable broth or water
- Salt to taste

For the Garnish:

- Fresh lemon wedges
- Fresh parsley, chopped

Instructions:

1. Marinate Chicken:
   - In a bowl, whisk together olive oil, soy sauce, minced garlic, dried oregano, paprika, salt, and black pepper.
   - Add chicken chunks to the marinade, coating them evenly. Let it marinate for at least 30 minutes.
2. Prepare Quinoa:
   - In a saucepan, combine quinoa and vegetable broth (or water).

o Bring to a boil, then reduce heat to low, cover, and simmer for 15-20 minutes or until quinoa is cooked and liquid is absorbed.

3. Preheat Grill:

   o Preheat your grill or grill pan to medium-high heat.

4. Assemble Kabobs:

   o Thread marinated chicken, bell peppers, zucchini, red onion, and cherry tomatoes onto skewers, alternating ingredients.

5. Grill Kabobs:

   o Grill the kabobs for about 10-15 minutes, turning occasionally, until the chicken is cooked through and the vegetables are charred and tender.

6. Fluff Quinoa:

   o Fluff the cooked quinoa with a fork.

7. Serve:

   o Serve the Grilled Vegetable and Chicken Kabobs over a bed of quinoa.

   o Garnish with fresh lemon wedges and chopped parsley.

Day 6:

Breakfast: Cottage Cheese and Berry Bowl

Ingredients:

- 1 cup cottage cheese
- 1/2 cup strawberries, sliced
- 1/2 cup blueberries
- 1/2 cup raspberries
- 1 tablespoon honey or maple syrup (optional, for drizzling)
- 1/4 cup granola
- Fresh mint leaves for garnish (optional)

Instructions:

1. Prepare Berries:

    ○ Wash and slice strawberries, and rinse blueberries and raspberries.

2. Assemble Bowl:

    ○ In a serving bowl, place a generous portion of cottage cheese.

3. Add Berries:

    ○ Arrange the sliced strawberries, blueberries, and raspberries on top of the cottage cheese.

4. Optional Sweetener:

    ○ If you prefer added sweetness, drizzle honey or maple syrup over the berries and cottage cheese.

5. Sprinkle Granola:

    ○ Sprinkle granola over the top for added crunch and texture.

6. Garnish (Optional):

    ○ Garnish with fresh mint leaves for a burst of freshness.

Lunch: Sweet Potato and Chickpea Buddha Bowl

Ingredients:

For the Sweet Potatoes and Chickpeas:

- 2 medium-sized sweet potatoes, peeled and cubed
- 1 can (15 oz) chickpeas, drained and rinsed
- 2 tablespoons olive oil
- 1 teaspoon ground cumin
- 1 teaspoon smoked paprika
- 1/2 teaspoon garlic powder
- Salt and black pepper to taste

For the Quinoa:

- 1 cup quinoa, rinsed
- 2 cups vegetable broth or water
- Salt to taste

For the Bowl:

- Mixed salad greens (e.g., kale, spinach, arugula)
- Avocado, sliced
- Cherry tomatoes, halved
- Red cabbage, shredded
- Tahini dressing or your favorite dressing

For Garnish:

- Sesame seeds
- Fresh cilantro, chopped

Instructions:

1. Roast Sweet Potatoes and Chickpeas:
   - Preheat the oven to 425°F (220°C).
   - In a bowl, toss sweet potato cubes and chickpeas with olive oil, ground cumin, smoked paprika, garlic powder, salt, and black pepper.
   - Spread them on a baking sheet and roast for 25-30 minutes or until sweet potatoes are tender and chickpeas are crispy.
2. Prepare Quinoa:
   - In a saucepan, combine quinoa and vegetable broth (or water).
   - Bring to a boil, then reduce heat to low, cover, and simmer for 15-20 minutes or until quinoa is cooked and liquid is absorbed.
3. Assemble Buddha Bowl:
   - In each bowl, arrange a bed of mixed salad greens.
   - Add a portion of roasted sweet potatoes and chickpeas, quinoa, sliced avocado, halved cherry tomatoes, and shredded red cabbage.
4. Drizzle with Dressing:
   - Drizzle your favorite dressing, such as tahini dressing, over the Buddha Bowl.
5. Garnish:
   - Garnish with sesame seeds and chopped fresh cilantro.

Snack: Roasted Chickpeas

Ingredients:

- 1 can (15 oz) chickpeas (garbanzo beans), drained and rinsed
- 1-2 tablespoons olive oil
- 1 teaspoon ground cumin
- 1 teaspoon smoked paprika
- 1/2 teaspoon garlic powder
- 1/2 teaspoon cayenne pepper (adjust to taste for spice)
- Salt to taste

Instructions:

1. Preheat Oven:
   - Preheat your oven to 400°F (200°C).
2. Dry Chickpeas:
   - Pat the rinsed chickpeas dry with a clean kitchen towel or paper towels. Removing excess moisture helps achieve crispiness.
3. Season Chickpeas:
   - In a bowl, toss the chickpeas with olive oil, ground cumin, smoked paprika, garlic powder, cayenne pepper, and salt. Ensure the chickpeas are evenly coated.
4. Spread on Baking Sheet:
   - Spread the seasoned chickpeas in a single layer on a baking sheet lined with parchment paper.
5. Roast in the Oven:
   - Roast in the preheated oven for 25-35 minutes, shaking the pan halfway through, until the chickpeas are golden brown and crispy.
6. Cool and Enjoy:
   - Allow the roasted chickpeas to cool on the baking sheet. They will continue to crisp up as they cool.
7. Serve:

- Once cooled, transfer the roasted chickpeas to a bowl and serve as a crunchy and flavorful snack.

Dinner: Tomato Basil Soup with Grilled Cheese Sandwich (using whole-grain bread)

Ingredients:

- 2 tablespoons olive oil
- 1 onion, chopped
- 2 cloves garlic, minced
- 2 cans (28 oz each) whole peeled tomatoes
- 1 cup vegetable broth
- 1 cup fresh basil leaves, chopped
- Salt and black pepper to taste
- 1/2 cup heavy cream (optional, for creaminess)
- Fresh basil leaves for garnish

Instructions:

1. Sauté Aromatics:
   - In a large pot, heat olive oil over medium heat. Add chopped onion and sauté until softened, about 5 minutes. Add minced garlic and cook for an additional 1-2 minutes.
2. Add Tomatoes:
   - Pour in the whole peeled tomatoes, breaking them up with a spoon. Include the juice from the cans.
3. Simmer:
   - Add vegetable broth and chopped basil. Bring the soup to a simmer. Season with salt and black pepper to taste.
4. Blend Soup:

- Use an immersion blender to blend the soup until smooth. Alternatively, transfer the soup in batches to a blender and blend until smooth. Be cautious when blending hot liquids.

5. Add Cream (Optional):
   - Stir in heavy cream if you desire a creamier soup.

6. Adjust Seasoning:
   - Taste and adjust salt and pepper as needed.

7. Garnish and Serve:
   - Garnish with fresh basil leaves and serve the Tomato Basil Soup hot.

Grilled Cheese Sandwich:

Ingredients:

- Whole-grain bread slices
- Butter
- Cheddar cheese slices

Instructions:

1. Assemble Sandwich:
   - Place cheddar cheese slices between two slices of whole-grain bread to form a sandwich.

2. Butter and Grill:
   - Butter the outsides of the bread slices.
   - In a skillet over medium heat, grill the sandwich on each side until the bread is golden brown, and the cheese is melted.

3. Serve:
   - Cut the grilled cheese sandwich into halves or quarters.

Day 7:

Breakfast: Buckwheat Pancakes with Fresh Strawberries

Ingredients:

- 1 cup buckwheat flour
- 1 tablespoon sugar
- 1 teaspoon baking powder
- 1/2 teaspoon baking soda
- 1/4 teaspoon salt
- 1 cup buttermilk
- 1 large egg
- 2 tablespoons melted butter or oil
- Fresh strawberries, sliced (for topping)
- Maple syrup (for drizzling)

Instructions:

1. Prepare Dry Ingredients:
   - In a large bowl, whisk together buckwheat flour, sugar, baking powder, baking soda, and salt.
2. Mix Wet Ingredients:
   - In a separate bowl, whisk together buttermilk, egg, and melted butter or oil.
3. Combine Wet and Dry Ingredients:
   - Pour the wet ingredients into the dry ingredients and stir until just combined. Do not overmix; a few lumps are okay.
4. Rest the Batter:
   - Let the batter rest for about 10 minutes. This allows the buckwheat flour to absorb the liquid.
5. Heat Griddle or Pan:
   - Preheat a griddle or non-stick pan over medium heat.
6. Cook Pancakes:
   - Spoon the batter onto the griddle to form pancakes. Cook until bubbles form on the surface, then flip and cook the other side until golden brown.
7. Repeat:
   - Continue cooking pancakes until all the batter is used.

8. Serve:

   - Stack the buckwheat pancakes on a plate.

9. Top with Fresh Strawberries:

   - Arrange fresh strawberry slices on top of the pancake stack.

10. Drizzle with Maple Syrup:

   - Drizzle maple syrup over the pancakes and strawberries.

Lunch: Spinach and Artichoke Stuffed Chicken Breast with Steamed Broccoli

Ingredients:

For the Stuffed Chicken Breast:

- 4 boneless, skinless chicken breasts
- Salt and black pepper to taste
- 1 cup fresh spinach, chopped
- 1/2 cup artichoke hearts, chopped
- 1/2 cup cream cheese
- 1/2 cup grated Parmesan cheese
- 2 cloves garlic, minced
- 1 tablespoon olive oil

For the Steamed Broccoli:

- **4 cups broccoli florets**
- Salt to taste
- Lemon wedges (optional, for serving)

Instructions:

Preheat Oven:

1. Preheat your oven to 375°F (190°C).

Prepare Chicken Breast:

2. Cut a pocket into each chicken breast by slicing horizontally, being careful not to cut all the way through.

3. Season the inside and outside of each chicken breast with salt and black pepper.

Make the Spinach and Artichoke Filling:

4. In a skillet, heat olive oil over medium heat.

5. Add minced garlic and sauté until fragrant.

6. Add chopped spinach and cook until wilted.

7. Stir in chopped artichoke hearts, cream cheese, and grated Parmesan. Cook until the cheese is melted and the filling is well combined.

Stuff Chicken Breasts:

8. Stuff each chicken breast with the spinach and artichoke mixture.

Bake:

9. Place the stuffed chicken breasts on a baking sheet.

10. Bake in the preheated oven for 25-30 minutes or until the chicken is cooked through.

Steam Broccoli:

11. While the chicken is baking, steam the broccoli. Place broccoli florets in a steamer basket over boiling water and steam for about 5 minutes or until tender-crisp. Season with salt.

Serve:

12. Once the chicken is done, serve it with steamed broccoli on the side.

13. Optionally, squeeze lemon wedges over the broccoli for added freshness.

Snack: Dark Chocolate and Almonds

Ingredients:

- 1 cup dark chocolate chips or chunks
- 1 cup whole almonds

Instructions:

1. Melt Chocolate:
   - In a heatproof bowl, melt the dark chocolate using a double boiler or by microwaving in 30-second intervals, stirring between each interval until smooth.

2. Coat Almonds:
   - Add whole almonds to the melted dark chocolate. Stir until all almonds are evenly coated.
3. Spoon onto Parchment Paper:
   - Using a spoon, scoop out clusters of chocolate-coated almonds and place them onto a parchment paper-lined tray. Ensure they are separated for easy removal later.
4. Chill:
   - Place the tray in the refrigerator for at least 30 minutes or until the chocolate has hardened.
5. Break Apart:
   - Once the chocolate is fully set, break the clusters apart into individual chocolate-covered almonds.

Dinner: Vegetable Barley Soup with a Side of Mixed Greens

Ingredients:
- 1 cup pearl barley, rinsed
- 1 tablespoon olive oil
- 1 onion, diced
- 2 carrots, diced
- 2 celery stalks, diced
- 3 cloves garlic, minced
- 8 cups vegetable broth
- 1 can (15 oz) diced tomatoes
- 1 cup green beans, chopped
- 1 cup corn kernels (fresh or frozen)
- 1 teaspoon dried thyme
- 1 teaspoon dried rosemary
- Salt and black pepper to taste

- Fresh parsley, chopped (for garnish)

Instructions:

1. Cook Barley:

    ○ In a separate pot, cook the pearl barley according to package instructions. Set aside.

2. Sauté Vegetables:

    ○ In a large soup pot, heat olive oil over medium heat. Add diced onion, carrots, celery, and minced garlic. Sauté until vegetables are softened.

3. Add Broth and Tomatoes:

    ○ Pour in the vegetable broth and add the diced tomatoes with their juice. Bring the mixture to a simmer.

4. Add Barley and Vegetables:

    ○ Add the cooked barley, green beans, corn, dried thyme, and dried rosemary to the pot. Stir well.

5. Simmer:

    ○ Allow the soup to simmer for 20-25 minutes or until the vegetables are tender.

6. Season:

    ○ Season the soup with salt and black pepper to taste.

7. Garnish:

    ○ Garnish with chopped fresh parsley.

Mixed Greens:

Ingredients:

- Mixed salad greens (e.g., spinach, arugula, romaine)
- Cherry tomatoes, halved
- Cucumber, sliced
- Balsamic vinaigrette or your favorite dressing

Instructions:

1. Assemble Salad:

- In a large bowl, toss together the mixed salad greens, cherry tomatoes, and cucumber.

2. Dress Salad:
   - Drizzle the salad with balsamic vinaigrette or your preferred dressing. Toss to coat.

Serve:

3. Serve Vegetable Barley Soup hot with a side of Mixed Greens.

Meal Preparation Tips:

1. Batch Cook: Prepare larger quantities of grains (quinoa, brown rice) and proteins (chicken, salmon) to use in multiple meals.

2. Chop Veggies in Advance: Wash, peel and chop vegetables at the beginning of the week for quick and easy meal assembly.

3. Pre-Portion Snacks: Divide snacks like mixed nuts, trail mix, and roasted chickpeas into portion-controlled containers for convenience.

4. Make-ahead Soups and Stews: Cook soups and stews in batches, portion them and store them for ready-to-heat meals during the week.

5. Prep Smoothie Ingredients: Portion and freeze smoothie ingredients in advance for quick blending in the morning.

6. Marinate Proteins: Marinate meats in advance to enhance flavor and reduce prep time before grilling or baking.

7. Stock Healthy Condiments: Keep healthy condiments like olive oil, balsamic vinegar and herbs on hand for easy flavoring.

COOKING TECHNIQUES FOR A NO GALLBLADDER DIET

1. Baking: Use this method for veggies and lean proteins like chicken or fish. It takes very little more fat.

2. Grilling: Grilling adds a great flavor to meats and vegetables without using a lot of oil. Marinate proteins in herbs and spices to increase flavor.

3. Steaming is a mild cooking method that keeps nutrients intact. Steam vegetables, fish, or chicken with as little fat as possible.

4. Sautéing with Broth or Water: For a lighter option, instead of using oil or butter, sauté veggies or proteins in a tiny amount of broth or water.

5. Roasting: Roasting vegetables or lean meats in the oven can bring out flavors without using too much oil. Season with herbs and spices.

6. Poaching is the gentle cooking of food in a simmering liquid. It's great for fish or poultry since it keeps them moist without adding fat.

7. Slow Cooking: Use a slow cooker to prepare soups, stews, and lean meats. This method produces tasty foods without requiring continual care.

8. Pressure Cooking: Using a pressure cooker, you may swiftly cook grains, legumes, and meats without using a lot of fat.

9. Broiling: Like grilling, broiling is a high-heat cooking method that may provide a lovely sear to proteins while using minimum fat.

10. Stir-Frying with Little Oil: When stir-frying, use a nonstick pan and little oil. Include a variety of colorful veggies as well as lean proteins.

11. Herb & Spice Infusion: Use herbs, spices, garlic, and onions liberally in your foods to add flavor without adding fat.

12. Homemade Broths: You may manage the fat content by making your own broths for soups and stews with lean meat, veggies, and herbs.

13. Adjust portion sizes to minimize overeating, as larger meals might be difficult to digest in the absence of a gallbladder.

14. Healthy Fats: When it comes to fats, choose healthier options like olive oil or avocado oil in moderation.

15. Acidic Ingredients: To add acidity to meals, use citrus juices or vinegar, which can enhance flavors without relying on excessive fats.

DINING OUT STRATEGIES

1. Examine the Menu in Advance:

Before you go, look over the restaurant's menu online to select suitable options and arrange your order.

2. Proteins can be grilled or baked:

   Proteins that are grilled, baked, or roasted, such as chicken, fish, or lean cuts of meat, are easier to digest.

3. Dressings and sauces on the side can be requested:

   Request dressings and sauces on the side so you can control how much you add to your dish.

4. Choose Lean Protein Sources:

   To reduce fat intake, choose lean protein sources such as poultry, fish, or plant-based choices.

5. Vegetables and fruits should be prioritised:

   To boost fibre and nutrients, prioritise vegetable-based foods and incorporate fruits in salads or as side dishes.

6. Stay away from fried and greasy foods:

   Avoid deep-fried and oily foods, which can be difficult to digest without a gallbladder.

7. Make Your Own Order:

   Don't be afraid to customise your meal by requesting changes that correspond to your dietary requirements.

8. Select Whole Grains:

   As a healthier carbohydrate source, choose whole grains such as brown rice, quinoa, or whole-grain pasta.

9. Inquire About Cooking Methods:

   Inquire about the culinary procedures used by the restaurant. Instead of frying, opt for grilled, baked, or steamed foods.

10. Keep Hydrated:

    To help digestion, drink water during the meal. Limit your intake of sugary or fizzy beverages.

11. Limit your alcohol intake:

Limit your alcohol consumption because it can sometimes aggravate intestinal discomfort.

12. Keep Portion Sizes in Mind:

To avoid overeating, pay attention to portion sizes and consider sharing dishes or taking leftovers home.

13. Choose Dairy Carefully:

To reduce the influence on digestion, choose low-fat or lactose-free dairy products.

14. Inquire about gluten-free options:

If you are gluten intolerant, ask about gluten-free options or replacements.

15. Pay Attention to Your Body:

Take note of how your body reacts to various foods. If you are uncomfortable, make a note of your options for future reference.

NAVIGATING RESTAURANT MENUS

1. Begin with lean protein:

Look for recipes that include lean proteins like grilled chicken, turkey, fish, or tofu.

2. Options for grilling or baking:

To avoid extra fats, choose grilled, baked, or roasted foods instead of fried foods.

3. Dishes that are vegetarian or vegetable-centric:

Investigate vegetarian or vegetable-centric alternatives, which are frequently lower in fat and higher in nutrients.

4. Grain Whole:

For a more nutritious carbohydrate source, choose recipes made with whole grains such as brown rice, quinoa, or whole-grain pasta.

5. Request sauces and salad dressings on the side:

Request sauces and dressings on the side to limit your consumption. Use these with caution.

6. Creamy sauces and soups should be avoided:

Avoid creamy sauces and soups since they might be heavy in fat and difficult to digest.

7. Limit High-Fat Dairy Consumption:

If you must have dairy, try low-fat or lactose-free varieties to reduce the impact on digestion.

8. Keep Portion Sizes in Mind:

To keep your intake under control, consider splitting dishes or ordering appetizer-sized amounts.

9. Inquire About Cooking Methods:

Inquire about the techniques used to prepare various foods. Grilled or sautéed is preferable to deep-fried.

10. Be Wary of Spicy Foods and Spices:

Spices should be avoided since some people find spicy foods difficult to digest. If necessary, choose milder choices.

11. Select Fruits and Vegetables:

In order to gain fiber and important nutrients, including fruits and vegetables in your order.

12. Make Your Own Order:

Don't be afraid to tailor your order to your dietary requirements. Most establishments are willing to work with you.

13. Hydrate yourself with water:

To help digestion, drink water during the meal. Limit your intake of sugary or fizzy beverages.

14. Inquire about gluten-free options:

If you are gluten intolerant, ask about gluten-free options or modifications.

15. Pay Attention to Your Body:

Take note of how your body reacts to various foods. If a specific item causes you distress, think about avoiding it in the future.

www.ingramcontent.com/pod-product-compliance
Lightning Source LLC
Chambersburg PA
CBHW070827250726
48662CB00003B/1113